JumpStart

MCAT

JumpStart MCAT

Chirag Amin, M.D.

University of Miami School of Medicine
Class of 1996
Resident, Orthopaedic Surgery
Orlando Regional Medical Center
Orlando, Florida

Vikas Bhushan, M.D.

University of California, San Francisco, School of Medicine
Class of 1991
Diagnostic Radiologist
University of California, Los Angeles, Medical Center
Los Angeles, California

Tao Le, M.D.

University of California, San Francisco, School of Medicine
Class of 1996
Resident, Internal Medicine
Yale-New Haven Hospital
Yale University School of Medicine
New Haven, Connecticut

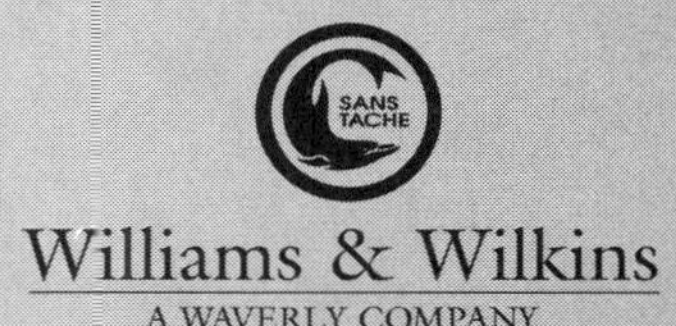

Williams & Wilkins
A WAVERLY COMPANY
BALTIMORE • PHILADELPHIA • LONDON • PARIS • BANGKOK
BUENOS AIRES • HONG KONG • MUNICH • SYDNEY • TOKYO • WROCLAW

Editor: Elizabeth Nieginski
Managing Editor: Alethea H. Elkins
Development Editor: Beth Goldner
Production Coordinator: Danielle Hagan
Designer: Ashley Pound Design
Cover Designer: Ashley Pound Design
Typesetter: Maryland Composition
Printer: Port City Press, Inc.
Binder: Port City Press, Inc.

351 West Camden Street
Baltimore, Maryland 21201-2436 USA

Rose Tree Corporate Center
1400 North Providence Road
Building II, Suite 5025
Media, Pennsylvania 19063-2043 USA

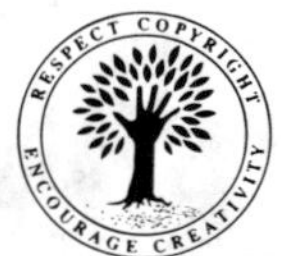

Printed in the United States of America

First Edition,

Library of Congress Cataloging-in-Publication Data
Amin, Chirag.
JumpStart MCAT : a high-yield student-to-student guide / [authors, Chirag Amin, Vikas Bhushan].
p. cm.
ISBN 0-683-18058-4
1. Medical colleges—United States—Entrance examinations—Study guides. I. Bhushan, Vikas. II. Title.
R838.5.A46 1996
610'.76—dc20

95-48460
CIP

The publishers have made every effort to trace the copyright holders for borrowed material. If they have inadvertently overlooked any, they will be pleased to make the necessary arrangements at the first opportunity.

To purchase additional copies of this book, call our customer service department at **(800) 638-0672** or fax orders to **(800) 447-8438.** For other book services, including chapter reprints and large quantity sales, ask for the Special Sales department.

Canadian customers should call **(800) 268-4178,** or fax **(905) 470-6780.** For all other calls originating outside of the United States, please call **(410) 528-4223** or fax us at **(410) 528-8550.**

Visit Williams & Wilkins on the Internet: **http://www.wwilkins.com** or contact our customer service department at **custserv@wwilkins.com.** Williams & Wilkins customer service representatives are available from 8:30 am to 6:00 pm, EST, Monday through Friday, for telephone access.

97 98 99
1 2 3 4 5 6 7 8 9 10

Dedication

To our teachers, who dedicated their time to providing us with knowledge and understanding.

To our colleagues and fellow premedical students, whose input, suggestions, and perspectives have been invaluable.

To our families, friends, and loved ones, who have provided us with their love and support throughout this endeavor.

Contributors

Radhika Sekhri-Breaden, M.D., M.P.H.
Resident, Internal Medicine
Stanford University

Stephen Gomperts
University of California, San Francisco
School of Medicine
Medical Scientist Training Program

Alexander Grimm
St. Louis University School of Medicine
Class of 1999

Sana Khan, M.D., Ph.D.
Resident, Diagnostic Radiology
University of California, Irvine

Ross Levine
Johns Hopkins University
School of Medicine
Class of 1998

Yi-Meng Yen
University of California, Los Angeles
School of Medicine
Medical Scientist Training Program

Associate Contributors

Julie Angulo
University of Miami
Class of 1994

Sameer Bhushan
University of California, Irvine
Class of 1996

Philip Galante
University of California, San Francisco
Hormone Research Institute

Parag Mathur
University of California, Berkeley
Class of 1997

Hoang Nguyen
Northwestern University
School of Medicine
Medical Scientist Training Program

Adrianne Gibbs-Phagan
University of Miami School of Medicine
Class of 1998

Uzma Samadani
University of Illinois, Chicago
Medical Scientist Training Program

Sunil Singhania
Pomona College of Osteopathic Medicine
Class of 1999

Vipal Soni
University of California, Los Angeles
School of Medicine
Class of 1999

contents

Part II High-Yield MCAT Facts

Foreword

Becoming a physician is viewed by many undergraduates as one of the few careers in which employment, satisfaction, and prestige remain secure. As a result, the pool of medical applicants has mushroomed over the past seven years. The number of matriculating premedical undergraduates has steadily risen and since 1990, there has been a 59% increase in the number of applicants. There are now more than three applicants for each available position in a medical school. The increased competition for admissions into medical school directly affects the number of students taking the Medical College Admissions Test (MCAT) and the need for them to perform well.

The MCAT is a formidable obstacle for most aspiring physicians. It is a stressful one-day test with 204 multiple-choice questions and two essays. All students applying to United States and Canadian medical schools must take the MCAT. A candidate's MCAT score and grade-point average (GPA) are the two most important factors determining medical school admission. There is a great deal of test-taking fear and anxiety surrounding the MCAT. Although most premedical students have experience with standardized tests, such as the Standardized Achievement Test (SAT) and the American College Testing assessment (ACT), the MCAT is usually their first encounter with a major multiple-choice marathon.

When preparing for the MCAT, students tend to overwhelm themselves, which prevents them from focusing on their studying efforts and the most relevant material. Many students simply do not have the testing savvy, proper strategies, and correct advice to successfully face this strenuous experience and, thus, commonly commit the following errors:

- "Stressing out" because of an inadequate understanding of the MCAT
- Becoming overwhelmed by the length and detail of review material
- Studying material that is rarely tested on the MCAT
- Buying the wrong review books or buying too many books
- Choosing an inappropriate commercial review course
- Using study methods that are inefficient, inappropriate, or outdated

JumpStart MCAT is a unique student-to-student guide designed to help premedical students quickly and effectively prepare for the MCAT. It includes advice on key issues, including study methods, MCAT format, and score results and interpretations. It also includes compact summaries of the key topics in all four science disciplines tested on the MCAT (i.e., biology, general chemistry, physics, and organic chemistry) and independent critical student evaluations of the major MCAT commercial review courses, review books, and sample exam books.

This practical guide emphasizes efficient study techniques, anxiety reduction, humor, and maximum exam performance for the time invested. In a concise manner, it presents topics, equations, and concepts that are most likely to appear in the science disciplines. Furthermore, we critically assess all the major review and exam preparation books currently on the market and recommend those to buy and those to avoid. We also provide concise summaries of the major commercial review courses.

The authors and Williams & Wilkins wish to regularly update *JumpStart MCAT*, so that this book continues to reflect the current material covered on the MCAT, which, like the field of medicine, is constantly evolving. If you have any helpful comments, strategies, high-yield facts, mnemonics, book reviews, or course reviews for the next edition, please use the forms in the How to Contribute section of this book to submit your contributions. Any student who submits material that we subsequently use will receive personal acknowledgment in the next edition of *JumpStart MCAT*.

Happy studying, and good luck!

Preface

This book is a unique, concise review guide to help aspiring medical students prepare for the MCAT. The contributor team includes medical students who have performed exceptionally well on the current MCAT. This book provides the reader with important advice on key issues needed for MCAT success. The book is divided into five major parts:

Part I provides you with an orientation to the MCAT. Our goal is to make you more familiar with the format of the MCAT and to help you organize your preparation for the exam. Knowing the specific details pertaining to the MCAT will help you feel more comfortable with the exam.

Part II provides a concise review of the most important facts you need to know for the MCAT. We believe that if you know and understand these topics, you will have the basic knowledge needed to perform well on the MCAT.

Part III reviews the many MCAT review books currently on the market. With the help of numerous independent student evaluations, we have evaluated these books specifically for their applicability for the MCAT. We looked at numerous criteria in evaluating these review books, including the quality and accuracy of the questions and explanations, readability, length, quality and number of visual aids (i.e., tables, diagrams), and cost. We hope our reviews make your search for resources easy and quick.

Part IV focuses on the commercial MCAT review courses that are available to students. We have summarized the key features of each review course, including information about cost, and hours of classroom instruction. Although we do not recommend a review course for every student preparing for the MCAT, students who want a more structured study environment and learn better from lectures may benefit from this information.

Finally, **Part V** briefly discusses the medical school application process. We provide insight on various steps in the application process, including advice on writing your personal statement, soliciting letters of recommendation, and the medical school interview. We provide you with guidance, from a student perspective, about what to expect and prepare for after taking the MCAT.

We hope you find this book useful and that it makes preparing for the MCAT easier for you. We greatly appreciate any comments, suggestions, or criticisms that you may have (see How to Contribute on page xxi). We look forward to receiving your input for future editions. Best of luck on the MCAT!

About the Authors

Chirag Amin, MD, recently graduated from medical school at the University of Miami and has started his residency training in orthopaedic surgery at Orlando Regional Medical Center. Chirag has been involved extensively in teaching and writing books. During medical school, he was an MCAT instructor for a national MCAT review course. As a co-author of *First Aid for the USMLE Step 1*, he led a major revision of the high-yield facts database. After residency, Chirag plans to pursue fellowship training in hand surgery.

Vikas Bhushan, MD, recently completed residency training in diagnostic radiology at the University of California, Los Angeles. His interest in medical education led to his development and publication of the highly successful *First Aid for the USMLE Step 1* in 1992. He is active in medical informatics and radiology research. Vikas earned his MD with Thesis from the University of California, San Francisco.

Tao Le, MD, recently earned his degree from the University of California, San Francisco School of Medicine, and he is now a resident physician in internal medicine at Yale-New Haven Hospital. Tao has been involved in several major writing and editing projects during the past five years. His latest book projects include the medical student guides *First Aid for the Match* and *First Aid for the Wards.*

Acknowledgments

This book would not have been possible without the encouragement and support of many people. We gratefully acknowledge the thoughtful comments, corrections, and suggestions of the numerous premedical students, medical students, and faculty who have supported the authors in developing this book. Special thanks to the Staff at Williams & Wilkins—Elizabeth Nieginski, Jane Velker, Tim Satterfield, Danielle Hagan, Kevin Thibodeau, Christopher O'Callaghan, and Beth Goldner—for their helpfulness and understanding. Also, we would like to thank especially Yi-Meng Yen, for his expert assistance with the diagrams and illustrations in this book. Other individuals who provided assistance and support include David Bard, Madhu Chopra, Andrea Fellows, Johnie Kelly, Jonathan Kirsch, Babak Kosari, Hao Le, Thong Le, Marc Mickiewicz, Ray Moloney, Vik Panchal, Rosina Samadani, Susan Sutliffe, and Alfred Sein. All of these individuals enthusiastically contributed to this work and have our sincere appreciation.

Chirag Amin
Vikas Bhushan
Tao Le

How to Contribute

JumpStart MCAT was created from the contributions and experiences of many students who successfully completed the MCAT. We invite you to participate in this process. Please send us your suggestions for mnemonics, diagrams, and test strategies as well as personal ratings and comments on review books that you used. The preferred way to submit corrections or suggestions is via electronic mail addressed to:

Chiragamin@aol.com
Vbhushan@aol.com
Taotle@aol.com

For MCAT news, updates, and corrections, visit our Internet Website at:

http://www.s2smed.com

Otherwise, please send entries, neatly written, typed, or on disk (Microsoft Word) to JumpStart MCAT, 720 Orange Street, #2, New Haven, CT 06511. You can also use the contribution forms on the following pages.

Contribution Form

Name: ______________________________

School/Affiliation: ______________________________

Address: ______________________________

____

Telephone: ______________________________

Cool tips, mnemonics, strategies, and corrections

Did you take a commercial MCAT review course? If so, which one? What was your overall assessment? Please comment on the quality of the review material, the classroom instruction, price, and the other resources at the review centers. Would you take the course again?

What student-to-student advice would you give someone preparing for the MCAT?

How else would you improve *JumpStart MCAT*? Any other comments or suggestions? What did you like most about the book?

Attach additional sheets if necessary. Thanks for your help!

(fold here)

Return Address

____

____

____

Postage required

Attn: Contributions
JumpStart MCAT
720 Orange Street, #2
New Haven, CT 06511

(fold here)

Book Reviews

Name: ______________________________

School/Affiliation: ______________________________

Address: ______________________________

____

Telephone: ______________________________

We need your feedback to help us rate and evaluate MCAT books for future students. Please comment on the MCAT books that you used below. Rate the books with a letter grade (e.g., A^+, B, C^-).

Title/Author/Publisher: ______________________________

Grade: __________ Time requirement: __________

Pros: ______________________________

____

Cons: ______________________________

____

Title/Author/Publisher: ______________________________

Grade: __________ Time requirement: __________

Pros: ______________________________

____

Cons: ______________________________

____

Title/Author/Publisher: ______________________________

Grade: __________ Time requirement: __________

Pros: ______________________________

____

Cons: ______________________________

____

Title/Author/Publisher: ______________________________

Grade: __________ Time requirement: __________

Pros: ______________________________

____

Cons: ______________________________

____

Photocopy this form if necessary. Thanks for your help!

(fold here)

Return Address

____

____

____

Postage required

Attn: Contributions
JumpStart MCAT
720 Orange Street, #2
New Haven, CT 06511

(fold here)

exam preparation

A Stop Worrying!

THIS BOOK IS intended to make your Medical College Admissions Test (MCAT) studying and preparation easier, more efficient, and less stressful. By helping you understand more about the MCAT, we will help you get the most out of your exam preparation. You are already familiar with taking science courses which require that you memorize large amounts of information in a short period of time. In addition, you have already taken standardized examinations such as the Scholastic Aptitude Test (SAT), the American College Testing Program (ACT), and various achievement tests. When preparing for the MCAT, however, you may become overwhelmed, which prevents you from focusing on your study efforts and the most relevant material. Typical errors that students make when approaching the MCAT include:

- "Stressing out" due to an inadequate understanding of the MCAT
- Starting to study too late
- Studying material that is rarely covered by the MCAT
- Not buying the right review books or buying too many books
- Leaping into a review course before looking
- Using study methods that are inefficient, inappropriate, or outdated
- Not understanding how the American Association of Medical College (AAMC) scores the MCAT or how MCAT scores affect an applicant's chances for admission

This book contains advice on how to avoid these common mistakes, thus helping you get the most out of your studying. First, however, you must understand the format and content of the MCAT.

1 WHAT IS THE MCAT?

MCAT scores and GPA are the two most important factors in your application.

The MCAT is a 1-day test that includes three multiple-choice sections and two essays. It is taken by all students applying to United States and Canadian medical schools, as well as by many applying to osteopathic and chiropractic schools. The exam is given only in the United States and Canada. The exam is administered twice a year, once in April and once in August. More than 36,000 students took the MCAT in August 1994 (Table 1-1), a number which has risen considerably over the past several years. In general, a medical school candidate's grade-point average, MCAT scores, and interview are the most important factors influencing medical school admission committees that make acceptance decisions.

2 HOW DO I SIGN UP FOR THE MCAT?

The MCAT is administered and scored by the Educational Testing Service under the guidance of the Association of American Medical Colleges (AAMC). In 1995, the cost of the examination was $150. A fee reduction is available for eligible individuals, lower-

The number of students applying to medical school is increasing, whereas the percentage of applicants accepted into medical school is declining.

TABLE 1-1. How Many People Take the MCAT?

Test Date	Students Taking the MCAT	Students Applying to Medical School	Students Accepted to Medical School
April 1991	22,408	29,243	17,206
September 1991	31,098		(59%)
April 1992	25,700	33,301	17,436
September 1992	32,841		(52%)
April 1993	27,968	37,410	17,464
September 1993	34,208		(47%)
April 1994	27,500	42,808	17,362
August 1994	36,240		(41%)
April 1995	30,059	45,365	17,317
August 1995	37,377		(38%)

ing the cost of the MCAT examination to $55; see "Is the MCAT Expensive?" (Part I A 3) for details. Current registration packets include an application (registration) card together with all current MCAT testing information. The packets should be available each February at your college's premedical advisory offices, as well as at local commercial test preparation centers. You can also get the packet by mail by phoning or writing:

MCAT Program
P.O. Box 4056
Iowa City, IA 52243
(319) 337-1357

Register early to get your favorite site.

You must register for the MCAT at least 1 month before the examination date. However, you should register to take the MCAT as soon as possible; if you register late, you may not get the testing site you want. More than one premedical student has had to rent a car and hotel room to take the MCAT at some out-of-the-way site. You should visit different testing sites near your residence or college, especially if your college is not an MCAT site. If the test-taking environment is important to you, we recommend that before registering, you familiarize yourself with the lecture hall, seating arrangements, cafeteria, and so forth.

3 IS THE MCAT EXPENSIVE?

You may qualify for an MCAT fee reduction.

Yes and no. In terms of the $40,000 to $100,000 you might have spent on your undergraduate education, the cost of the MCAT and the medical school application process is a drop in the bucket. On the other hand, preparing thoroughly for the MCAT ends up costing more in money and time than most students initially estimate. You will spend $150 to register for the MCAT, $100 to $300 on review books, and possibly another $500 to $800 on a review course. For this reason, **invest your time and money carefully in review books and courses.** Consult our review (Parts III and IV) for advice about the best books and courses for your money. If you can demonstrate financial need, you may apply for the $55 MCAT reduced registration fee [a form is included with the

MCAT application, or you can request an MCAT fee reduction form by calling AAMC student services at (202)828-0060]. Some review courses also offer a discount for students who are receiving financial aid; contact course administrators for details.

You should also keep in mind that the application process for medical schools gets more expensive from here on. You will be expected to pay $15 to $30 for each school you check off on your American Medical Colleges Admission Service (AMCAS) application, as well as $50 to $100 for each secondary application and each non-AMCAS application. Again, the same fee reduction or waiver process exists for these application fees; consult the AMCAS application for additional information. Furthermore, students are expected to pay for travel (plane, hotel, car) expenses associated with medical school interviews (unless you apply to certain combined graduate-degree programs). Never mind that medical school can cost upward of $150,000 for the 4 years.

4 WHEN SHOULD I TAKE THE MCAT?

If you are planning to apply to medical schools during your senior year, take the MCAT in either August or April of your junior year: **the year before you apply to medical school** (Figure 1-1). The advantage of the August date is that it could give you a school-free summer in which to focus solely on preparing for the MCAT. If you opt to take the test in April, you will allow yourself more time to finish requisite and supplementary course work for the MCAT, but you may have less time for MCAT preparation—depending on your academic course load. Other students taking the MCAT in April are also taking courses at this time, however; you are not at a disadvantage. Consider taking a light spring-semester course load.

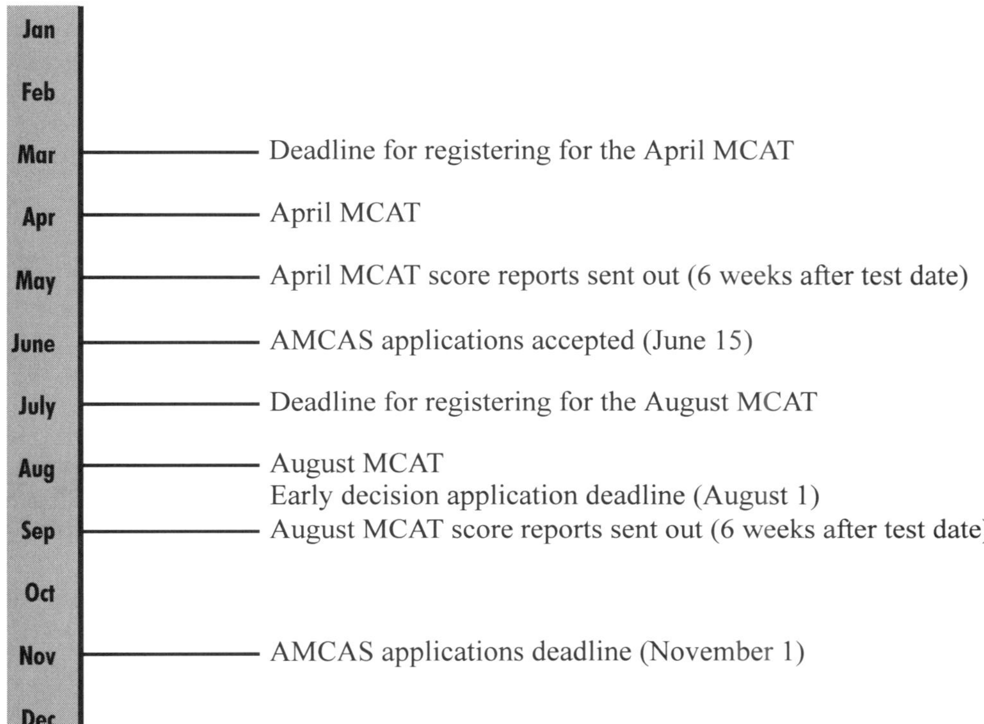

Figure 1-1. Premedical MCAT flowchart and timeline.

In any case, avoid taking the test prematurely. *Do not take the MCAT until you have finished all the requisite course work* (see Part I E 1). You can take the April MCAT while finishing one or two (not three) required science courses, but you will have to cover the later material in these courses on your own before taking the MCAT. In addition, some medical schools prefer that all their applicants' MCAT scores be from the same time period so they can accurately compare applicants (most schools will accept MCAT scores only taken in or after 1992; consult the AAMC *1996–97 Medical School Admissions Requirements* for details).

Timing the MCAT is critical.

More important, avoid taking the MCAT in the fall of the year that you plan to apply to medical school (i.e., August of your senior year). Most medical schools interview and select candidates for admission on a rolling basis, meaning that they begin interviewing and accepting students with scores from previous MCAT sessions before the AAMC releases the August MCAT scores to the medical schools. Far too many qualified medical students have been rejected or put on a waiting list by all the medical schools to which they applied—because they postponed taking the MCAT.

5 WHAT SHOULD I BUY RIGHT AWAY?

Purchasing these three publications is a must!

Even before you register for the MCAT, you should order the three sets of publications made available by the AAMC. The first set contains the *MCAT Student Manual* and *MCAT Practice Test 1,* and it costs approximately $15. The second set of publications contains *MCAT Practice Items* and *MCAT Practice Test 2* and also costs approximately $15. *MCAT Practice Test 3* is the latest offering from the AAMC, and costs approximately $15. These publications offer the only real MCAT questions available for your test preparation.

The fourth book for your shelves is a copy of the current *Medical School Admission Requirements,* another publication written by the AAMC, which gives admissions information and application deadlines for all medical schools in the United States and Canada. This publication also contains useful information for minority applicants as well as for high school students who plan to apply to combined college and medical school programs. All these books can be found in most undergraduate bookstores, or they can be purchased by writing or calling:

Membership and Publication Orders
Association of American Medical Colleges
2450 N. Street, NW
Washington, DC 20037-1129
(202) 828-0416

B What Is the Format of the MCAT?

THE MCAT HAS four major sections: verbal reasoning, physical sciences, writing sample, and biological sciences. All sections are multiple choice except the essay section, and they contain both passage-based and discrete multiple-choice questions. Each multiple-choice question has four choices. In the three sections, you are allotted an average of 78

MCAT Test Day		
	Registration & Seating	*Approximately 1 hour*
	Verbal Reasoning	*65 questions in 85 minutes*
	Break	*10 minutes*
	Physical Sciences	*77 questions in 100 minutes*
	Lunch	*1 hour*
	Writing Sample	*2 essays in 60 minutes*
	Break	*10 minutes*
	Biological Sciences	*77 questions in 100 minutes*

Figure 1-2. Format of MCAT administration.

seconds per question. The writing sample section contains two essays that are to be completed in 60 minutes (Figure 1-2).

1 VERBAL REASONING

The verbal reasoning section includes 8 to 11 passages on various subjects from the humanities (e.g., literature and history), the social sciences (e.g., sociology and anthropology), and the natural sciences (e.g., astronomy, geology, and paleontology). Each passage is followed by 6 to 10 related questions. Therefore, this section mainly tests your ability to understand each passage, to evaluate the material within that passage, and to use this material to answer the questions posed.

2 PHYSICAL SCIENCES

The physical sciences section tests your ability to understand and apply concepts from physics (50%) and inorganic chemistry (50%). Therefore, this section mainly tests your ability to understand and evaluate the material within each passage, then use this information to answer the questions posed. Approximately 62 of the 77 questions refer to 10 to 11 passages. You are expected to answer these questions using both the information you read in the passage and your general knowledge of physics and inorganic chemistry; many passages include graphs and tables that you are expected to interpret and apply. Each passage is followed by 5 to 10 questions. The remaining questions—approximately 15—are not based on the written passages.

3 WRITING SAMPLE

See Part II B for high-yield facts that will help you master the essay.

The writing sample section of the MCAT requires that you write two independent essays. You are given one-half hour (timed separately) for each essay question, during which time you are expected to write a well-organized, persuasive, legible, and error-free essay developed around a central idea. You are not expected to have any specific knowledge of the essay topic. Instead, for each essay, the AAMC will present you with a statement, and you are expected to do the following:

- Explain what the statement means.
- Describe a specific situation in which the statement does **not** hold true.
- Discuss what you think determines when the statement holds true and when it does not.

4 BIOLOGICAL SCIENCES

Unlike the physical sciences section in which physics and general chemistry weigh equally, the biological sciences section contains more biology (65%) than organic chemistry (35%).

The biological sciences section tests your ability to understand and apply concepts from biology (65%) and organic chemistry (35%). Approximately 62 of the 77 questions are based on 10 to 11 passages, with each passage followed by 5 to 10 questions. (The remaining questions—approximately 15—are not based on passages.) You are expected to answer these questions using both the information in the passage and your general knowledge of biology and organic chemistry; in addition, many passages include graphs and tables that you are expected to interpret and apply.

C Scoring

1 HOW IS THE MCAT SCORED?

There is no penalty for guessing. *Do not leave any answers blank!*

In each section except the writing sample, your raw score is based on the number of questions you answer correctly. *There is no penalty for guessing.* Fill in all answer spaces. Your raw score is then converted to a scaled score between 1 and 15, with 1 being the lowest and 15 the highest. The only scores you receive will be between a 1 and 15 for each multiple choice section and a letter score for the essay portion of the examination. The AAMC will not tell you how many questions you answered correctly or incorrectly. However, the AAMC will provide the percentile of your scaled score. The percentile explains what fraction of students achieved a comparable or a lower score than you.

Although premedical students often perceive some sections (e.g., physical sciences) as tougher than others, the AAMC scales the distribution of scores to a standard distribution, with a mean of 8.0 and a standard deviation of 2.5 for each section. This figure is determined by adjusting the raw-score to scaled-score conversion scales (Figure 1-3). In addition, each examination administration uses a slightly different conversion scale, sometimes resulting in no scores in the 14 to 15 or 1 to 2 range on a particular section. This effect occurs more often with the verbal reasoning scores than with the biological science or physical science scores.

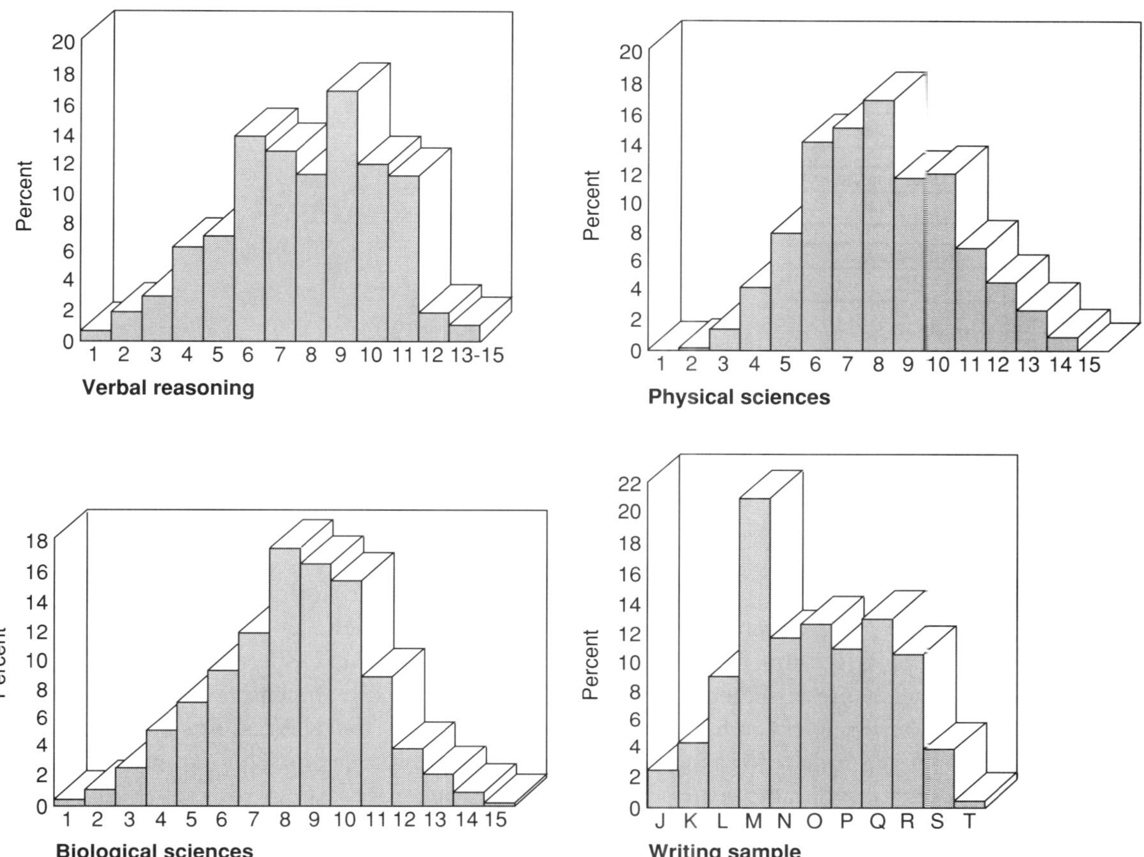

Figure 1-3.
Distribution of MCAT scores (combined April and August 1995). *Percent* = percent achieving scores.

The writing sample section of the MCAT is scored differently from the other three sections.

The writing samples are scored on the basis of their overall quality with no separate evaluations on organization, content, grammar, coherence, fluency, or other essay-writing criteria. Each essay is evaluated by two readers. After reading an essay, each reader independently assigns it a score based on a scale of 1 (lowest) to 6 (highest). The final essay score averages the two readers' scores. If these scores vary by more than one point, a third reader evaluates the essay in question to determine the final score. The final essay scores for both essays are then combined and converted into a letter score ranging from J (lowest—equivalent to a total of 2 points) to T (highest—equivalent to a total of 12 points).

To help you understand how the MCAT is scored and how scores are distributed, a sample score report with distribution information for the combined April and August 1995 MCAT administrations is included as Figure 1-4. Look at the score distribution in Figure 1-3; notice how many people score within 1 standard deviation of the mean (8 ± 2.5).

2 WHO GETS THE SCORES?

Although medical school admission committees do look at other factors, your grade-point average (GPA) (both science and overall), your MCAT score, and your interviews are the most important factors determining whether you will be admitted to medical school. In their efforts to sift through the large number of candidates who apply to med-

APRIL 1994

TEST (SCALED) SCORES			
VERBAL REASONING	PHYSICAL SCIENCES	WRITING SAMPLE	BIOLOGICAL SCIENCES
9	9	Q	9

SEX	DATE OF BIRTH	STATE OF RESIDENCE
M	9/6/69	CA

SOCIAL SECURITY NUMBER	AMCAS RELEASE
999-99-9999	YES

Your scores have been sent to these coded non-AMCAS schools as requested on your answer document.

999 999 999 999 999 999

©1994 Association of American Medical Colleges

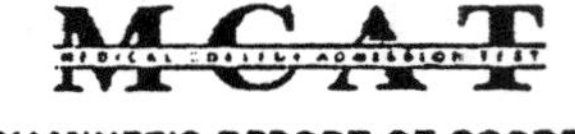

EXAMINEE'S REPORT OF SCORES

MCAT Program Office
P.O. Box 4056
Iowa City, Iowa 52243
Telephone: (319) 337-1357

99999

John Doe
999 MCAT Street
Over Here, AA 99999

This report will not be accepted by a medical school. You must have an official AAMC MCAT test report forwarded to the medical school by AMCAS

Figure 1-4.
Sample MCAT score report.

ical school each year, some schools use a "formula" based on student grades and MCAT scores to determine which candidates will be interviewed.

Given this formula, grades and MCAT scores **can** offset each other. The formula usually uses a sliding scale; that is, a high GPA can compensate for low MCAT scores. Conversely, if you have lower grades, extremely high MCAT scores can dramatically improve your chances in the medical school admissions process. Nevertheless, the most successful applicants possess both high grades and good MCAT scores, so you should work hard on both.

Some schools use "cutoffs"; that is, they require a specific minimum score on the MCAT, GPA, or both before inviting you for an interview. As a result, the remainder of your application often cannot offset low grades or low MCAT scores, no matter how many hours you volunteered in the emergency room or how well you performed in intramural sports.

3 WHAT DO I NEED TO SCORE ON THE MCAT?

When you begin preparing for the MCAT, you must set realistic numerical goals. The MCAT is the only objective measure by which the medical school admission committees can compare students from different schools; therefore, the test is especially pivotal if you come from a lesser known or smaller school. In fact, for many students the MCAT score is the most vital component of the medical school application because it reflects a student's most recent academic performance. It is usually taken as a sign of academic progress or, on the down side, regression. For example, getting a C, then B+, and then a 13 in physical sciences may be perceived as continuing improvement, whereas an A– and B+ followed by a 6 may be perceived as a negative trend.

Before studying for the MCAT, set rough numerical goals for yourself on each section. First, see Table 1-2, which lists the available average MCAT scores and grades for the 1995 entering classes from the 126 medical schools in the United States. The data come from several sources, including the *1996–97 Medical School Admissions Requirements,* published by the AAMC. If you really want to go to a particular medical school and your grades are somewhat lower than the mean GPA associated with that school, aim to score above their published MCAT mean. In 1994, more than 72% of

TABLE 1-2. GPA/MCAT Average Scores for American Medical Schools

School	Science GPA	Non Science GPA	Overall GPA	Biological Sciences	Physical Sciences	Verbal Reasoning	Mean Score	% Matriculated In-State Applicants
ALABAMA								
Alabama			3.55	9.7	9.4	9.9	9.7	79.0
Alabama, South			3.60	9.3	9.1	9.4	9.3	90.6
ARIZONA								
Arizona			3.50					100.0
ARKANSAS								
Arkansas			3.52					97.9
CALIFORNIA								
Stanford			3.60	11.0	11.0	10.0	10.7	50.0
Loma Linda			3.57					57.2
California, U of								
Davis								100.0
Irvine	3.55		3.58				10.2	100.0
Los Angeles (UCLA)	3.57	3.64						92.3
San Diego			3.62					95.9
San Francisco		3.72	3.71	11.0	11.0	11.0	11.0	77.8
California, Southern			3.47	10.0	10.0	10.0	10.0	87.3
COLORADO								
Colorado			3.70				9.9	84.1
CONNECTICUT								
Connecticut			3.50				9.7	85.2
Yale								9.0
DISTRICT OF COLUMBIA								
George Washington			3.40					1.9
Georgetown			3.51					2.7
Howard								9.8
FLORIDA								
Florida			3.66				9.3	98.3
Miami			3.56	9.5	9.2	9.5	9.4	90.7
Florida, South	3.70	3.70	3.70	9.8	9.6	9.5	9.6	99.0
GEORGIA								
Medical College of								98.9
Mercer								100.0
Morehouse								64.7
Emory			3.62	9.9	9.7	9.9	9.8	48.3
HAWAII								
Hawaii			3.44	9.6	9.3	9.6	9.5	82.1
ILLINOIS								
Illinois, U of								93.4
Illinois, Southern								98.6
Chicago—Pritzker	3.48		3.51				10.2	45.2
Northwestern			3.51				75th percentile	48.3
U Health Sci Chicago			3.20					28.7
Loyola—Stritch			3.47					50.8
Rush								90.8

Continued

TABLE 1-2. GPA/MCAT Average Scores for American Medical Schools—Cont.

School	Science GPA	Non Science GPA	Overall GPA	Biological Sciences	Physical Sciences	Verbal Reasoning	Mean Score	% Matriculated In-State Applicants
INDIANA								
Indiana			3.59	9.4	9.4	9.4	9.4	91.4
IOWA								
Iowa	3.60		3.60	9–10	9–10	9–10	9–10	88.0
KANSAS								
Kansas							60th percentile	92.6
KENTUCKY								
Kentucky			3.44					87.5
Louisville			3.50					91.2
LOUISIANA								
Louisiana State								
New Orleans	3.40							100.0
Shreveport	3.40		3.40					100.0
Tulane			3.50					14.9
MARYLAND								
Maryland			3.50				9.0	82.8
Johns Hopkins								12.7
Uniformed Services, Health Sciences			3.40				9.8	N/A
MASSACHUSETTS								
Massachusetts	3.50							100.0
Harvard			3.70	11.3	11.3	10.5	11.0	12.5
Boston								34.5
Tufts								27.4
MICHIGAN								
Michigan, U of			3.60					64.9
Michigan State								83.6
Wayne State			3.50					92.2
MINNESOTA								
Minnesota, U of								
Duluth			3.44	9.0	8.7	9.0	8.9	88.0
Minneapolis			3.55					91.9
Mayo			3.67	10+	10+	10+	10+	14.3
MISSISSIPPI								
Mississippi			3.60					100.0
MISSOURI								
Missouri, U of								
Columbia	3.50		3.60					97.9
Kansas City								69.7
Saint Louis			3.61	10.0	9.9	9.8	9.9	32.5
Washington	3.76	3.79	3.77					8.1
NEBRASKA								
Nebraska			3.64					97.5
Creighton	3.45		3.56					9.8

Continued

TABLE 1-2. GPA/MCAT Average Scores for American Medical Schools—Cont.

School	Science GPA	Non Science GPA	Overall GPA	Biological Sciences	Physical Sciences	Verbal Reasoning	Mean Score	% Matriculated In-State Applicants
NEVADA								
Nevada			3.4				9.6	71.2
NEW HAMPSHIRE								
Dartmouth								13.6
NEW JERSEY								
UMDNJ—New Jersey Medical School			3.35					89.4
UMDNJ—Robert Wood Johnson			3.47					87.7
NEW MEXICO								
New Mexico			3.40				8.9	93.2
NEW YORK								
SUNY								
Brooklyn								90.0
Buffalo								99.3
Stony Brook								92.0
Syracuse								93.1
Columbia								32.0
Cornell	3.53			10.5	10.5	10.5	10.5	39.6
New York University								50.9
Rochester								36.7
Albany			3.50					42.8
Albert Einstein								44.1
Mount Sinai			3.50					58.3
New York Medical								23.0
NORTH CAROLINA								
UNC Chapel Hill								93.1
East Carolina			3.35	8.3	7.7	8.4	8.1	100.0
Duke								32.0
Bowman Gray of Wake Forest								51.9
NORTH DAKOTA								
North Dakota	3.53		3.55	8.9	8.6	8.7	8.7	67.3
OHIO								
Cincinnati								83.3
Medical College of	3.28		3.37	9.2	8.9	8.7	8.9	81.8
Northeastern (NEOUCOM)								95.1
Ohio State			3.50					79.5
Wright State								86.7
Case Western Reserve			3.50				10.0	65.4
OKLAHOMA								
Oklahoma			3.55					87.7
OREGON								
Oregon Health Sciences			3.60					83.9

Continued

TABLE 1-2. GPA/MCAT Average Scores for American Medical Schools—Cont.

School	Science GPA	Non Science GPA	Overall GPA	Biological Sciences	Physical Sciences	Verbal Reasoning	Mean Score	% Matriculated In-State Applicants
PENNSYLVANIA								
Penn State			3.50					52.3
Temple	3.40						10.0	62.1
Pittsburgh			3.52				10.4	59.3
Pennsylvania, U of			3.60				10–11	23.3
Thomas Jefferson	3.40						9.9	44.4
Medical College of								50.4
Hahnemann								47.4
RHODE ISLAND								
Brown								14.1
SOUTH CAROLINA								
Medical University								82.9
South Carolina, U of								95.9
SOUTH DAKOTA								
South Dakota	3.60	3.67	3.63					86.0
TENNESSEE								
Tennessee State, East			3.40	8.8	8.6	9.1	8.8	85.0
Tennessee, Memphis			3.50	9.0	9.0	9.0	9.0	91.5
Vanderbilt								13.7
Meharry								10.0
TEXAS								
Baylor			3.60					65.9
Texas, U of								
Houston			3.41					86.6
San Antonio			3.58					87.4
Dallas (Southwestern)								85.4
Galveston			3.50					90.5
Texas A & M			3.63					100.0
Texas Tech								96.7
UTAH								
Utah								74.0
VERMONT								
Vermont			3.30				8.9	38.5
VIRGINIA								
Virginia, U of			3.56				85th percentile	70.5
Medical College of			3.40				9.7	68.8
Eastern Virginia								62.0
WASHINGTON								
Washington			3.58	10.3	10.0	9.9	10.1	91.0
WEST VIRGINIA								
Marshall			3.50					93.9
West Virginia			3.55	8.8	8.5	8.6	8.6	90.9
WISCONSIN								
Medical College of								52.1
Wisconsin								79.7
OUTSIDE THE U.S.								
Ponce			3.30					68.3
Puerto Rico	3.39		3.50	7.0	7.0	6.0	6.7	96.3
U Central del Caribe			3.11					90.0

students entering medical school had cumulative GPAs of 3.26 or above. Also, keep in mind that the published means include minority students; you should consider the data in Table 1-3 when evaluating your GPA and MCAT scores.

From reviewing Table 1-2, you can generalize: If you want to get into a highly competitive public or private medical school, plan on obtaining MCAT scores of at least 10 to 12 on each section while maintaining a GPA of 3.5 to 3.7. On the other hand, if you are interested in attending one of the less competitive public schools, you may get by with MCAT scores of 9, 10, or higher. In the case of the less competitive private schools, you probably need to obtain scores of 9 to 11, or higher. However, because many of the highly competitive schools do not release their GPA/MCAT information, you should not rely on published score reports alone. Furthermore, out-of-state students should consider not applying to medical schools that have not accepted any out-of-state applicants (e.g., UC Davis, Mercer, LSU-Shreveport). Perhaps the best advice is to speak to senior premedical students from your undergraduate college about their experiences to get a better understanding of admissions standards.

Few schools give their average scores on the essay (writing sample) section, thereby making it even harder to judge what essay score you need to get into medical school. In general, the essay section is not weighed as heavily as the other three sections. However, you should still take this section seriously (see Part I B 3, C 1); a below-average score on this section will harm your chances for gaining admission into medical school. In addition, medical schools can (and occasionally do) request copies of applicants' essays.

The essay section gets less weight than the other three sections.

To help refine your MCAT goals, take a diagnostic MCAT test (one with a 1 to 15 scale) at least 2 months before the actual MCAT administration. You can use your practice scores to gauge your workload for the following months.

- If you miss your target on all sections, do not despair; many people improve dramatically after intensive preparation. You should, however, plan on spending the bulk of your time in the following months preparing for the MCAT.
- If your performance is uneven and if you score more than 1 to 2 points below your goal on a particular section, plan on spending a lot of time on that particular area.
- If you hit the bull's-eye, raise your expectations—the higher your score, the better your chances of being admitted to the school of your choice.

4 SHOULD I RETAKE THE MCAT?

If your MCAT scores do not meet your expectations and you are willing to invest many more months studying, retaking the exam is an option. Do not be intimidated or discouraged by your first set of scores. Remember that the MCAT is a 1-day examination, and **anyone** can have a bad day. If your scores are inconsistent with your college grades (see Table 1-2), or with your practice scores, you definitely should consider retaking the exam.

Before you decide to try again, however, be aware that medical schools will weigh your second score more strongly than your first, which means that you **can** redeem yourself with a markedly better MCAT performance the second time around. Thus, you want to ensure that you can at least match your first set of scores, if not improve them. In fact, medical schools assume that students who retake the MCAT will do better the second time; **AAMC research shows that people who retake the MCAT improve approximately 1 point overall without additional preparation**. Your goal in retaking the MCAT should be to increase your score by at least 2 points.

If you decide to retake the test, use the experience you gained from your first MCAT test.

In addition, when you retake the MCAT, you are usually not as enthusiastic or motivated as you were the first time around. Therefore, obtaining the same level of MCAT proficiency or a higher level may involve considerably more effort and time. Use the experience gained from your first MCAT test to improve your level of preparedness the next time around.

5 SHOULD I APPLY TO MEDICAL SCHOOL EVEN IF I HAVE WEAK SCORES?

If you do poorly on the MCAT and you think that retaking the exam will not help, consider that some premed students with an 8 or less do get into medical schools in spite of their MCAT scores. Many medical schools use a "formula" or a cutoff based on a numerical combination of GPAs and MCATs, so a good GPA may compensate for weaker MCAT scores.

If your GPA is also borderline, you have two choices.

a. Improve your GPA as rapidly as possible.

Consider taking a number of easier classes, or classes without grade competition until you mail your application. You can even consider taking "graded independent study" or community-college courses to improve your GPA. Consult your adviser and successful premeds from your school.

b. Your file needs something that makes your application distinctive or exceptional.

For example, you could perform extraordinary volunteer work or community service, participate in a ground-breaking research experience, or become an all-American sports star.

6 SHOULD I RELEASE MY SCORES? IF SO, WHEN?

When you register to take the MCAT, you may elect to have your scores withheld. If you choose this option, you are the only one who will receive a copy of the scores. Then, should you choose to release your scores after you have evaluated them, you simply write a letter to the AAMC section for student services authorizing them to send your scores to the medical schools to which you have applied. The disadvantages of this option are that you give up your six free medical school reports and incur a 2-month delay in reporting your scores to medical schools. If you are taking the test late (say, in the fall of your senior year), this option should be dismissed.

D Minority and Foreign Students

1 WHAT IF I AM A MEMBER OF A MINORITY GROUP?

Many American medical schools have aggressive recruitment policies for underrepresented minorities. The AAMC defines "underrepresented minorities" as African Americans, Native Americans (American Indians and Alaskan natives), Mexican-Americans, and mainland Puerto Ricans. If you belong to one of these minorities, your GPA and MCAT scores might be slightly less important than discussed previously (Table 1-3). Other factors such as community service may be just as important. Consult the AAMC *1996–97 Medical School Admissions Requirements* for details.

TABLE 1-3. Profile of 1995 Applicants Accepted by Medical Schools

Variable	African American	Mainland Puerto Rican	Mexican American	Native American	Commonwealth Puerto Rican	Other Hispanic	White	Asian
Sci GPA	2.92	3.03	3.01	3.10	3.07	3.28	3.45	3.57
Non Sci	3.31	3.30	3.35	3.37	3.49	3.48	3.57	3.59
Cum GPA	3.09	3.15	3.16	3.22	3.26	3.38	3.5	3.51
VR	7.4	7.9	8.3	8.5	5.7	9.1	9.6	9.2
PS	6.9	7.6	7.8	7.4	6.7	8.7	9.4	10.1
BS	7.2	7.9	8.3	8.0	7.1	8.9	9.5	9.9
WS	O	O	O	O	N	O	O	O

2 WHAT IF I AM A FOREIGN STUDENT?

Most American medical schools require that foreign students attend college in the United States for at least 1 year—and even then, foreign students are not eligible for most financial aid (and sometimes must place their entire tuition in an escrow account before matriculating). Although foreign students often have difficulty gaining acceptance into American medical schools, it can be done. If you are a foreign student, you must perform extremely well on the MCAT (especially on the verbal reasoning and essay sections) and maintain your GPA. The best advice may come from talking with the few successful foreign applicants each year. Use your contacts to track them down.

E Course Work

1 WHAT COURSES DO I NEED FOR THE MCAT?

Make sure that, at a minimum, you have completed all of the required course work before you take the MCAT.

Focus on specific MCAT subject material while taking your premed courses.

The course work of the well-prepared MCAT student is similar to (but not the same as) that required for medical school admission (Table 1-4).

To prepare for the MCAT, you should take at least 1 year of biology with laboratory, including at least one semester of cellular/molecular biology and one semester of organismic/evolutionary biology. In addition, you should take 1 year of inorganic chemistry with laboratory, although you can get away with an accelerated one-semester course in inorganic chemistry if you had college-level or advanced placement chemistry in high school. You should also have at least one semester of organic chemistry with laboratory; the second semester of organic chemistry is usually required for medical school admission but is not necessary for the MCAT biological sciences section. Finally, 1 year of physics (preferably with laboratory) is necessary for the MCAT. **There is no calculus-based physics on the exam.**

Some schools offer special premed versions of the previously mentioned science courses, many of which focus on medical/biological applications of chemistry, physics, and math. These courses are an excellent idea, especially if your main interest in such subjects stems from having to take the MCAT and wanting to go to medical school. If you take the more rigorous classes, be prepared for the workload, and be aware that much of what you learn will be more advanced than the concepts you will use when taking the MCAT. Pay specific attention to subject material tested frequently on the MCAT.

Most schools also offer or require a semester of English composition or expository writing. You should take this course; not only is it required for most medical schools, but also it will help you refine your writing skills for the essay section of the MCAT. Finally, for the verbal reasoning section, you should read journal articles and books, both scientific and nonscientific, to bolster your reading speed and comprehension.

Supplemental course work is useful but not crucial for MCAT success. If you have the time, take a class in vertebrate or human physiology, because many of the passages, graphs, and tables in the biological sciences section are standard fare in a good physiology course. A course in biochemistry can also enhance your MCAT preparation, by familiarizing you with concepts that appear frequently on the MCAT (acids and bases,

TABLE 1-4. Undergraduate Courses for MCAT Preparation

Necessary	Supplementary	Optional
1 year biology: cellular/molecular biology organismic/evolutionary biology	Expository writing	Upper level mathematics
1 year inorganic chemistry	Second semester organic chemistry	Upper level physics
1 semester organic chemistry	Physiology	Human anatomy
1 year noncalculus-based physics	Biochemistry	Physical chemistry

metabolism, enzymes, and hormones). Finally, a course in speed reading, reading comprehension, and test-taking can help with the entire exam, especially if you are a slow reader and have a hard time finishing tests.

2 WHAT IF I'VE ALREADY GRADUATED FROM COLLEGE?

If you graduated from college without the necessary courses or with low grades in your science course work, a postbaccalaureate program may be right for you. These programs are designed for people with college degrees who need further course work before applying to medical school. Such programs normally offer the basic premedical requirements as well as supplemental advanced science courses. Students are expected to maintain a minimum grade-point average. If you fulfill their requirements, those who sponsor these programs will usually help you apply to medical school by writing letters of recommendation, reviewing your application, and in some cases preparing you for the MCAT (if not, consider taking a review course). In addition, some of these programs are specifically geared for underrepresented minorities and disadvantaged students.

If you enroll in one of these programs, expect to spend the bulk of your time studying for your classes. Since these programs typically last up to 2 years (and especially since many postbaccalaureate students are older), students are often tempted to take the MCAT early in their postbaccalaureate training, to accelerate the process of entering medical school. Unless your performance on the sample exams is awe inspiring, wait until you have finished **all** the necessary course work before taking the MCAT, even if it means waiting an extra year before going to medical school. In addition, consider taking advanced courses in physiology and biochemistry to further your MCAT preparation.

If you wish to continue your education while studying for the MCAT on your own, one good option is a Master's in Public Health (MPH) program. This type of program will broaden your perspective on medicine, and admission committees often consider an additional degree a favorable asset. Besides, this degree is respectable to add to an MD (i.e., MD, MPH), as opposed to doing research and getting a master's degree in science that you will rarely mention in the future. Getting a PhD is entirely different (and a lengthy) process.

F When Should I Start Preparing for the MCAT?

PREP TIME FOR THE MCAT varies among individuals. Following is a timeline that you can use in the weeks, months, and years before taking the MCAT.

1 YEAR BEFORE

The AAMC claims that "the scientific competency you will be expected to demonstrate on the MCAT is derived from basic principles and concepts in biology, general chemistry, organic chemistry, and physics." Therefore, first and foremost you should finish all of the required course work during the years leading up to the MCAT. Also consider supplemental course work like physiology and biochemistry to boost your MCAT preparation. Try to study MCAT material in parallel with your preparation for these courses—a strategy that should improve your grades along with your MCAT scores.

If you have one or more years before you plan to take the MCAT, you should also consider taking certain advanced science courses (see Part I E 1). Such courses can help you better understand basic scientific concepts by discussing them in more complicated contexts. Again, if you take the MCAT in April, plan a light spring semester to gain more time then to study for the MCAT.

Know your strengths and weaknesses in terms of the MCAT.

Before your urgent preparation for the MCAT begins, you should know your strengths and weaknesses in the material tested on the exam. Essentially, you should use this time to learn the basic sciences and other relevant material well the first time so you can minimize review time in the weeks before the MCAT; or if you are weak in the verbal reasoning or writing sample section, you can practice writing essays. Many schools offer writing tutorial courses on a pass/fail basis.

The MCAT stresses reading comprehension, not just a fund of knowledge. Read both scientific and nonscientific topics in the years before the exam. Read a variety of expository and opinion articles found in periodicals such as *Newsweek, Time, Scientific American, Journal of the American Medical Association,* and the *New England Journal of Medicine.* These articles will not only help you with the verbal reasoning section but also improve your ability to interpret and apply passages in the science sections. If you are a slow reader, consider taking a speed reading course. It will also help you with your medical school interviews; interviewers love well-informed and well-balanced candidates.

2 MONTH BEFORE

In the months preceding the test administration, register for the MCAT (see Part I A 2) and get the AAMC practice materials and student manual. Before registering for the MCAT, talk to people who have already taken the test to find out about test sites. Try for a favorable environment; the smaller the room and the fewer the number of students in that room, the more efficiently proctors can administer the test (and hence, the shorter the test). In addition, large desks help you organize your test materials, and spread-out seating provides an environment with fewer distractions. As mentioned earlier, if the testing environment is key for you, visit local testing sites, choose the site you like best, and register for the MCAT as soon as possible.

Plan to "peak" the day of the MCAT.

You should be studying seriously for the exam several months before the test date.

You should be studying seriously for the exam several months before the test date. At this time you should also decide about a commercial review course and buy the latest editions of MCAT review books. If you are bothered by family and friends who ask about your MCAT preparation and goals, do not tell them you are taking the MCAT (or do not tell them when you are taking it). You should also consider that preparing for the MCAT is like preparing for a race; you should peak the day of the MCAT. Accordingly, the months before the exam are a buildup to the "big day." Start by taking a few practice tests to identify your strengths and weaknesses before designing your preparation schedule. Then prepare a timeline that sets deadlines for the completion of certain topics and dates for practice tests. For the physical sciences and biological sciences sections, combine content review with practice tests, and for the verbal reasoning and essay sections, work through as many practice passages and questions as possible. If you doubt your ability to organize your exam preparation, or you need help with the subject matter, research and enroll in a reputable review course at least 2 months before the exam. Remember that you want to peak the day of the MCAT.

3 THREE WEEKS BEFORE

Building up your endurance is essential to MCAT success.

At this point, you should be completing your subject-by-subject review. For the next 2 weeks, you should concentrate on taking practice tests under simulated MCAT conditions. Have a friend time the sections for you, and start the test at 9 A.M. to get used to the time of day the MCAT is administered. If you finish a section early, **do not go on to the next section until time is up.** Building up your endurance is essential to MCAT success. Also, do not look at the answers to the test until you complete the entire practice test.

Most important, after each test, you should go through the answers and carefully analyze your mistakes. Keep a list of topics with which you have trouble, and consult science textbooks for additional information on these subjects.

4 ONE WEEK BEFORE

If you have already put in a lot of preparation time and are meeting your goals on the sample tests, take it fairly easy the last week before the MCAT. Do a full-length practice test under proctored conditions 1 week before the test date. If you are in a review course, the instructors will usually administer one MCAT under simulated testing conditions.

During the week, you should focus on going through practice passages, not on learning new material. The idea is to develop more test-taking stamina than you will need on the exam day. If you are really fanatical about the test, and you have little or no concurrent course work, you can try the following schedule:

- Early morning—practice verbal passages.
- Late morning—practice physical science passages.
- Noon—break for lunch.
- Early afternoon—write one or two essays.
- Late afternoon—practice biology passages.

If possible, try to adhere to the same basic daily schedule (start time and breaks) you will use on the test day. Try to wake up at the same time you plan to arise on the test day, and go to sleep at the same time you plan to go to bed the night before the exam. Remember that sleep deprivation has cumulative effects; a good night's sleep on the Thursday night before the test is as important as a good night's sleep on the Friday night before the test. If it is convenient, go to the test center and do these practice passages there. Each evening, you may also want to spend an hour going over the list of subjects that give you trouble. Analyze your "stupid" errors, and plan how to avoid them on the test day.

5 ONE DAY BEFORE

Relax.

If you have an established pattern that worked for previous examinations, keep it on this final day before the MCAT. Of greatest importance is to relax. Stress over the test is perfectly normal, but do not let it unnerve you. If you feel stressed, find something to keep your mind off the test; for example, go see a movie. Try not to study the day before the exam. If you must study, do not study new material; simply scan high-yield facts like those in this book. The night before the exam, set out five or six # 2 pencils and a few black pens, registration materials, two picture IDs, and a nonbeeping timer. You may also want to make lunch and snacks the night before to avoid food hassles the day of the exam.

G Day of the Exam

Arrive at the test center early.

TAKING THE EXAM is stressful enough. Plan the day in advance to avoid stress about anything else. A wake-up call helps. Eat a nutritious breakfast. Protein may enhance logical thinking capabilities; eat something more substantial than sugared cereal. Plan to arrive at the test center no later than 7:30 A.M. If you are using public transportation, have everything rehearsed, and allot sufficient time for delays.

If you get to the test center early and have free time, try to stay away from study material. Instead, read something light, such as newspapers, magazine articles, or maybe even practice passages. If you decide to do practice passages, however, do not answer the questions or look up their answers; the idea is to get into the right frame of mind for the verbal reasoning section and avoid using test time for warming up. This free time is also opportune for a trip to the bathroom.

1 ADMINISTRATIVE MECHANICS AND WHAT TO EXPECT ON THE TEST DAY

Before you get a seat assignment, the administrators will fingerprint you (think of it as prison for a day). Next the administrators give you an answer booklet for all the test sections, as well as endless standardized forms to fill out. Think of this stage as another test, this one a test in patience. Expect to spend up to an hour for fingerprinting, seating, and filling out administrative information in the answer booklet. At the beginning of every section, the administrators will hand out a question booklet for that section. At the end of every section, the administrators will collect the question booklet and the answer sheet, which you will tear out of the answer booklet. At this point, they will also check the name on your picture ID against the name on the answer sheet. Every time the proctors let you leave the room for a break or for lunch, they will ask to see your card on your return. All this distributing and collecting of materials prolong the length of the MCAT from 6 to almost 10 hours. Do not expect to finish early or even on time.

a. Morning Session

The test day is not the time to experiment with new techniques. For example, wear earplugs or use a nonbeeping timer only if these techniques have previously worked for you.

You should make full use of the 10-minute break after the verbal reasoning section. Visit the restroom even if you don't feel the urge. If you want a snack, stay away from candy bars. Snacks with complex carbohydrates (such as fruits and granola bars) provide the right amount of energy to pace yourself through the day.

b. Lunch

Lunch is your chance to regroup and replenish depleted energy supplies. Avoid talking about the test at this time, because the stress of this discussion can adversely affect your performance on the rest of the test. Do not take a nap after lunch. Bring your lunch to avoid depending on the cafeteria services or being subject to the unfortunate mishaps that can be associated with leaving the testing site. Avoid heavy or spicy foods.

c. Afternoon Session

During the second 10-minute break after the essay, go for a short walk or stretch. Now is the time to indulge in candy bars or other sweets. Research shows that a drop in subjective alertness is normal during the middle of the afternoon, although many students catch their "second wind" in the middle of the biological sciences section. If this happens to you, check your early answers for careless mistakes. Finally, if you finish the biological sciences section early, use the extra time to check your answers.

2 AFTER THE EXAM

As soon as you finish the MCAT, go out and celebrate. Remember that you have just finished one of the longest and most difficult exams you will ever face. And do not fret about your mistakes; the exam is over; no worrying or rethinking is going to change your score. If you are very concerned that you did poorly, you may want to debrief by analyzing the areas that gave you trouble and making notes on what to study if you retake the exam. Then, put these notes aside until the scores come out. Remember that the MCAT alone does not determine your success in applying to medical school and that these scores are not correlated with your degree of success or failure in medical school or in your medical career.

You can expect score reports in the mail within 6 to 8 weeks.

PART II

high-yield mcat facts

A Verbal Reasoning

1 TIME ALLOTMENT

Unlike the physical sciences and biological sciences sections, you cannot study specific content material for the verbal reasoning section. Proper preparation for this section involves lots of practice questions and passages. For this section, you are expected to answer 65 multiple-choice questions in 85 minutes, giving you an average of 1.3 minutes per question (not a lot of time). In addition, you must read the 8 to 11 passages on which the questions are based, which means that you have even less time available to answer each question. You should allot a little over 1 minute per question, a figure that includes the time to read the appropriate passage. According to this rule of thumb, for a seven-question passage you have 8 minutes to read the passage, then read and answer the questions. If you follow this time management strategy, you will have approximately 10 extra minutes for checking your answers after you finish the section or for finishing a difficult passage. Use the 8 minutes for 7 questions rule as a guideline to pace yourself both when you practice and when you take the actual test.

You cannot study specific content material for the verbal reasoning section.

2 RECOMMENDED APPROACHES TO VERBAL REASONING PASSAGES

Various approaches to a verbal reasoning passage follow.

- Critically read each passage in less than 2 minutes and then answer the questions. If you decide to use this approach, find ways to improve your reading comprehension and your efficiency in answering questions. Some test takers find it helpful to spend 10 to 15 seconds (no longer) scanning the passage before reading the entire selection. In this way, you can quickly identify the central thesis of the passage, the main ideas of each paragraph, and the direction or slant of the passage before you begin reading. Some people find that this technique reduces time spent reading and locating the answers to the questions within the passage.

2 minutes per passage.

- Read the questions first, read the passage, and then answer the questions. Some people find that knowing the questions gives them a good idea of what to look for in the passage, which saves time during the reading process. However, a majority of students find that this technique ultimately wastes more time. It is unlikely that you will remember all the questions while you are reading the passage, so you will have to read the questions again, anyway. Determine whether this technique saves you time when doing verbal reasoning passages; if not, stick with the first option.
- Other students prefer to mark the passage as they read, underlining or circling important ideas as they are presented. Briefly jot down in the margins one or two phrases summarizing each paragraph. It may also help to circle specific words that indicate a change of thought or idea (e.g., however, although). By glancing at your notations, you can quickly find relevant information to help

answer the questions. If this "landmark" technique improves comprehension and helps locate answers without slowing your progress or interrupting your train of thought, it is recommended. Beware: it is easy to go overboard. Nevertheless, with practice, annotations serve as a "conceptual map" that help you quickly locate the answers to the questions within the passage.

Annotating the passage helps to identify relevant information.

No matter which technique you choose, try all three first. The effectiveness of different reading techniques varies from person to person. Instead of blindly sticking to the strategy endorsed by your review course teacher, by Dr. Flowers, or by your mom, experiment when taking practice tests in the months leading up to the MCAT.

Another important fact is that you need no previous knowledge of the topics presented in the passages to answer the questions. On the other hand, familiarity with the topic of a particular passage can improve your speed and accuracy as long as you stick to the facts and arguments presented in the actual passage (rather than the facts and arguments as you remember them).

3 TYPES OF QUESTIONS USED BY THE AAMC

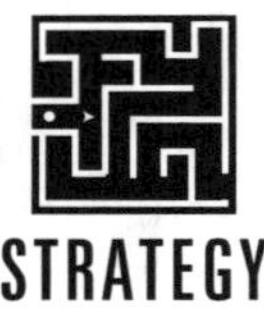

STRATEGY

Several types of questions regularly appear on the test.

Familiarity with the types of questions that the AAMC uses over and over should improve your speed, and therefore your score. For example, one type of question (usually beginning with "According to the passage") asks you to refer to a specific point in the passage. In this situation, go back to the passage, find the relevant statement, and answer the question. In another type of question, all the answer choices except one are true. Instead of looking for the three true answers, locate the one false response. Another type of question asks you to extrapolate or predict based on information presented by the author of the passage. Once again, the specific details you need to answer this question are located within the passage. Whatever the question type, **read each question carefully;** many students make mistakes because they overlook key words such as "except" or "never."

Quickly identify the main idea of the passage and each paragraph.

Another group of questions may ask about the main idea of a passage or a particular paragraph (usually beginning with "The purpose of the following paragraph is to ..."). Learn how to locate the central thesis of the passage as you read it; it is often at the beginning or the end of the reading selection. Similarly, most authors include headings or "tag" their paragraphs with introductory statements that help you identify the purpose of that section. Practice identifying the focus of each passage as you read; this skill will save you time on test day.

Finally, some questions ask about the tone or the opinion of the author. There is no set strategy you can use to determine the tone or bias of the author; however, the passage will contain salient remarks that signify the tone of the author (unless the tone is "objective"). Look for use of first person. Also, look for judgmental and evaluative words; for example, effective, efficient, undoubtedly, obviously, however, nevertheless, understandably.

4 PRACTICE

The most important part of verbal reasoning preparation involves practice, practice, and more practice. After you finish a series of practice passages, check your answers and **identify and evaluate your mistakes.** Go over your wrong answers; figure out why you missed those questions. Then tabulate and categorize your mistakes. In this way, you can identify consistent errors and work at eliminating them. With practice, you may be able to identify the answers within a passage before you even read the questions. Finally, remember to stick to the passage and try not to read between the lines.

Check your answers; identify and evaluate your mistakes.

5 RUNNING OUT OF TIME

If you are running out of time (i.e., if you have 5 minutes or less) and you have passages left to read, start answering the questions without reading the passage. Remember that the AAMC does not require students to choose an inflammatory, extreme, or improperly biased answer. Therefore, eliminate answers that state, "Native Americans were much more primitive than the colonists who replaced them" or "Doctors make way too much money." Cross out unreasonable answers, and then **take a guess for every question.** Following are two ways to avoid running out of time. First, when a particular passage gives you a lot of trouble, go to the next passage and return to the troubling passage at the end (but don't forget it). Second, fill in the answer sheet after each passage. Far too many students tell horror stories of botching entire sections by planning to fill in the entire answer sheet at the end of the section and then running out of time. Some test takers prefer not to fill out the answer booklet every single time they answer a question; instead, they mark the question booklet with the correct answer and then fill in all the correct answers ("batch fill-in") after each passage.

Answer every question; there is no guessing penalty!

B Writing Sample

1 GRADING

The essays that you write for this section of the MCAT are graded holistically (see Part I C for details). To ensure that 50,000 essays are graded in a reasonable amount of time (read $$$), readers evaluate each essay in no more than 90 seconds (yes, a mere minute and a half). Moreover, graders may be bored, aggravated, and tired by the time they reach your essay; they have been sitting in the same room reviewing essay after essay, minute after minute, for hours on end. In addition, they have probably read essays similar to yours many more times than you can imagine. None of the graders can maintain a high level of interest after reading 510 student essays on the same topic. You do not need dramatically original ideas to do well on your essay; even if you do, the readers may not even notice, given the pace they are keeping. Readers will base their grade on their "holistic" impression of your essay after glancing over it for approximately 1 or 2 minutes. Your job is to make their job as easy as possible.

Grading follows a holistic rather than analytic approach.

2 FIRST IMPRESSIONS

First impressions are the most important.

First, focus on how your essay looks at the superficial level. As a student you probably learned the old adage, "Quality over quantity." Temporarily forget what you have learned. This approach is fine when you have time, but the essay section is under strict time control. A lengthy essay (at least three pages long) makes a good first impression; it implies that you are fluent and comfortable with the English language. If it's too short, the graders may assume the worst. Second, avoid errors, but accept that your essay will not be all A+ rhetoric, because much of it may not even be read. First impressions are the most important, which is not only a rule of life but also a rule for the MCAT essay.

Cross out mistakes neatly.

Be neat. If you have messy handwriting, work on improving it. The excuse that MDs have poor handwriting carries no weight here, especially since the graders are not MDs. **Draw a neat single line through any mistake, place parentheses around it, and keep going.** (This method is the "medicolegally correct" way to fix errors in patient charts.) Some students have even used erasable ink. Once again, however, the main objective is to be neat.

3 ESSAY INSTRUCTIONS

Both essays present a statement and ask you to write a unified essay that includes the following topics.

a. Explanation

Explain what you think the statement means. The statement is usually expressed in absolute terms; that is, it contains words such as "always" or "never."

b. Description

Describe a specific situation in which the opposite of the statement is true.

c. Discussion

Discuss what you think determines when the statement is true or false.

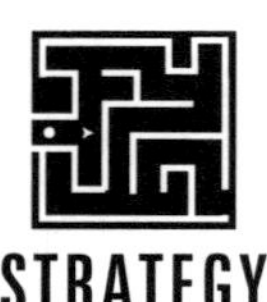

STRATEGY

Do exactly what the instructions say to do, and make it obvious that you are following the instructions. Answer each part of this question in a separate paragraph; start each paragraph with labeled "tag sentences" that show the grader what you will do in the following sentences. **Be sure to perform all three tasks;** if you do not, the best you can expect on the essay is a 3 (equivalent to an overall score of an "O").

4 RECOMMENDED APPROACHES TO THE ESSAY

Show the grader that you are a learned and well-read person. Use quotes from political figures, philosophers, and writers. Some students even memorize a handful of powerful, "versatile" quotations to pepper the essay. You can find books of quotations (e.g., *Bartlett's Familiar Quotations*). Remember a few general, all-purpose quotes, the kind you might use at a cocktail party to convey a scholarly and cultured image.

Quotations can add eloquence to your essay.

Save your big words and complex sentence constructions for the introductory and closing paragraphs and the topic sentences; if the grader is going to look closely at anything, it will be these sentences. Even though the readers are unlikely to scrutinize your examples, it cannot hurt to use worldly and academic references. Moreover, examples contribute to the length of the essay, so put as many as you can into your essay.

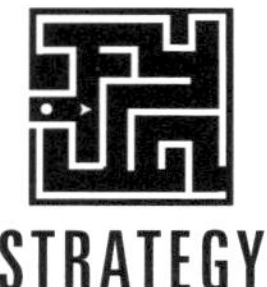

STRATEGY

The first and last sentences of a paragraph are the most important.

Finally, when practicing essay writing, aim primarily at becoming more fluent and performing the three tasks. You don't need to be an amazing writer. When you walk into the MCAT, you should be able to perform the necessary tasks and write a superficially intellectual essay on almost any topic, without much thought at all. Remember that the biological sciences section follows the essay section. Save your brain power and concentration for the "home stretch."

5 WRITING TIPS

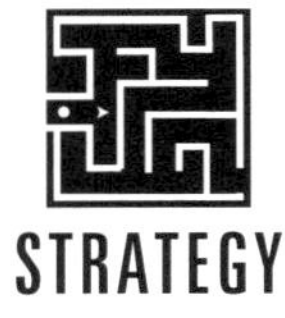

STRATEGY

- Be politically correct.
- Forget slang.
- Avoid repeating yourself in the essay (this concept may seem obvious, but is harder than you think, especially when only 5 minutes remain and you develop writer's block).
- Analyze rather than overexplain the topic.
- Write the essay as if you were writing an article for a newspaper. You want a sensational headline (first sentence) and closing line (last sentence) that leaves them thinking (puts the question in a new light).
- Favorite essay topics on the MCAT include the environment, politics, and philosophy. Familiarity with these topics is helpful as is understanding basic principles and fundamentals in these areas.
- Use a number of descriptive "action" words as well as imagery without going overboard to capture the reader's attention.

C Introduction to the Physical Sciences

The physical sciences section is difficult and thorough. Study hard and try to excel on this section of the MCAT.

AFTER FINISHING the verbal reasoning section, most students feel the effects of time pressure, but begin to relax during the first 15-minute break. Unfortunately, the physical sciences section comes next and hits the unprepared student like a sledgehammer. For many MCAT test takers, the physical sciences section is the most difficult section of the exam. In fact, the AAMC uses a more generous conversion curve for the physical sciences than it does for the other sections, meaning that you can get more questions wrong before your score goes down. In any case, the majority of medical schools admit students with slightly lower average physical sciences scores than their biological sciences and verbal reasoning scores, which means that most students get many physical sciences questions wrong. However, this dark cloud has a silver lining. You can do very well in relation to the other applicants without getting all of the questions right as long as you know how to prepare and practice for the physical sciences section.

Most students have difficulty finishing this section within the time allotted. Work quickly and efficiently.

In the physical sciences section, you must answer 77 questions within 100 minutes. Just as with the verbal reasoning section, you have 1.3 minutes per question. Once again, spend 1.25 minutes on each question (which will leave you a little extra time for answering hard questions and for checking your answers). Do not get bogged down on any one question or passage. Skip a passage that gives you a lot of trouble, and go back to it at the end. You can "batch fill-in" the answer sheet, but never go to the next passage without filling in the answers from the previous one. The MCAT has no guessing penalty, so answer every question, even those nasty electromagnetism ones!

Practice doing simple calculations in your head or by hand.

The AAMC states that the physical sciences section is evenly divided between inorganic chemistry and physics. When preparing for inorganic chemistry, focus on important chemical concepts, not on small details. Do not worry about memorizing the boiling point of ethanol; instead, understand why liquids boil and how boiling points change with intermolecular attraction and molecular weight. Instead of memorizing the gas laws, understand why the volume of a gas increases when you heat it at constant pressure. If you study inorganic chemistry concepts instead of memorizing fact after fact, you will do better on this section of the exam. Finally, practice doing simple calculations in your head or by hand, because you cannot use a calculator on the day of the test (your parents had to do it this way).

Practice quick calculations. You must be comfortable in estimating and performing calculations with numbers in scientific notation.

With the possible exception of organic chemistry, most premedical students fear the physics questions more than the questions from any of the other scientific disciplines. Do not fear this section; once again, concentrate on concepts, not on memorizing equations. The physics tested on the MCAT is not that difficult; a lot of it (especially mechanics) can be understood using common sense, especially gravity and kinematics. Know Newton's laws cold; they contain the most important principles of mechanics. Electricity and magnetism are a little more difficult; but once again, if you stress qualitative concepts, you will do fine. The passages will include many of the necessary details for answering the multiple-choice questions.

The questions and answers interspersed among the high-yield facts are strictly for understanding and content reinforcement, and they are very valuable for this purpose. However, they do not reflect the content, format, or difficulty of questions that appear on the actual MCAT exam.

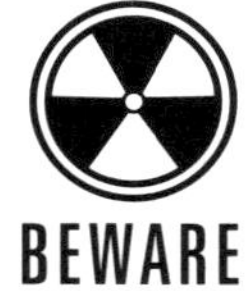

D Physics

1 KINEMATICS

Kinematics is the study of objects in motion with respect to space and time. In particular, kinematics is used when calculating parameters for the motion of an object, such as its velocity, acceleration, and distances traveled over a given period of time.

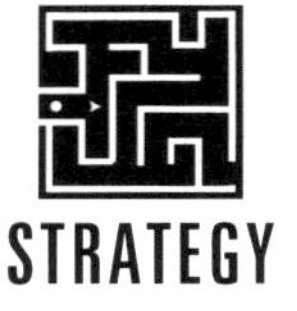

To do well on the physical sciences section of the MCAT, you must know the following very basic, very important equations cold. Practice doing problems with these formulas until they are second nature. You do not need to know calculus for the MCAT, so you can focus on these simple non–calculus-based formulas and ace the MCAT kinematics questions.

$$x = x_0 + v_0 t + \frac{1}{2} at^2$$

$$v = v_0 + at$$

$$v^2 = v_0^2 + 2as$$

a = acceleration (m/s^2)
s = distance traveled (m)
t = time (sec)

v = current velocity (m/s)
x_0 = initial position (m)
v_0 = initial velocity (m/s)
x = current position (m)

In addition, always estimate before you calculate your answer. For instance, assume that g = 10 m/s^2. Scan the answer choices to see how precise they expect your calculations to be.

A car has a constant acceleration, going from rest to 20 m/s in 5 seconds. How far does the car travel in that time?

ANSWER

First, calculate the acceleration of the car.

$$v = v_0 + at$$

$$20 = 0 + a \times 5$$

$$a = 4 \text{ m/s}^2$$

Then find the distance traveled.

$$x = x_0 + v_0 t + \tfrac{1}{2} at^2$$

$$x = 0 + 0 \times 5 + \tfrac{1}{2} \times 4 \times 5^2$$

$$x = 50 \text{ meters}$$

or

$$v^2 = v_0^2 + 2as$$

$$20^2 = 0^2 + 2 \times 4 \times s$$

$$400 = 8s$$

$$s = 50 \text{ meters}$$

QUESTION

The velocity of a particle is plotted over time as shown.

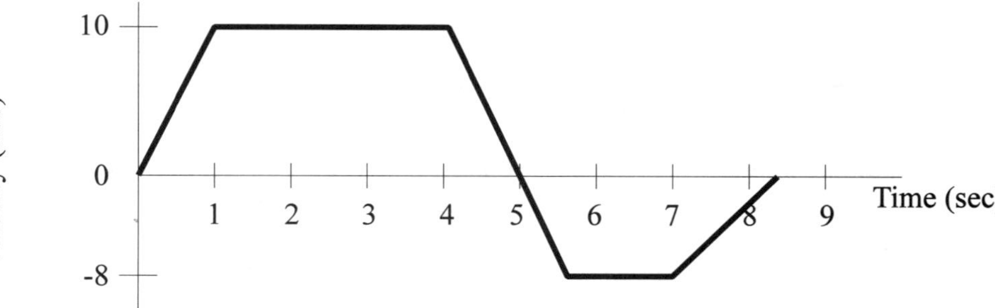

(a) How fast is the particle accelerating between 4 and 6 seconds?
(b) How far does the particle travel in the first 5 seconds?
(c) What is the net distance that the particle travels between 4 and 6 seconds?

ANSWER

To answer these graphic-interpretation problems, you must understand how to extract the necessary information from them. In general, the slope of a graph is equal to the change along the y-axis divided by the change along the x-axis.

In this situation:

$$slope = \frac{\Delta v}{\Delta t} = a$$

(a) The slope of the line between t = 4 and t = 6 seconds is:

$$\frac{-8 - 10}{6 - 4} = -9 \text{ m/s}^2$$

(i.e., acceleration is less than zero because the object is decelerating)

(b) To find the distance [i.e., the area under the curve (AUC)], either split this area into two triangles and a rectangle or remember the formula for the area of a trapezoid. For simplicity, solve for the area of a trapezoid.

$$Area = \frac{B + b}{2} h$$

B = length of the base of the trapezoid
b = length of the top of the trapezoid
h = height of the trapezoid

$$x(0 \rightarrow 5) = AUC(0 \rightarrow 5) = \frac{5 + 3}{2} \times 10 = 40 \text{ meters}$$

(c) This question is similar to the one in (b):

$$\text{Net } x = AUC(4 \rightarrow 5) + AUC(5 \rightarrow 6) = 5 + (-6) = -1 \text{ meter}$$

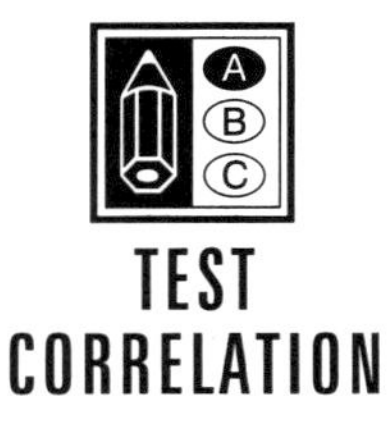

TEST CORRELATION

The physical sciences section on the MCAT contains many kinematics questions, both discrete and passage-based. Sometimes these questions are framed in terms of sound or light (e.g., How far or how fast has this sound/light wave traveled?), and you must use these kinematics equations in combination with the sound and light equations (see Part II D 9).

2 PROJECTILES

Projectile motion is the movement of an object in space with respect to its path of motion in both the vertical direction (y) and the horizontal direction (x). The path of motion, known as its trajectory, is always parabolic when gravity is involved. **You can maximize the distance traveled by a projectile by firing it at a 45-degree angle.**

$$v_x = v_0 \cos(\theta)$$
$$v_y = v_0 \sin(\theta)$$

v_x = velocity in the horizontal direction (m/s)
v_y = velocity in the vertical direction (m/s)
v_0 = initial speed of the object (m/s)
θ = angle between the vector v_0 and the horizontal plane

The x-component of velocity is used to find the total distance traveled. The y-component of velocity is used to find out how long the projectile was in the air.

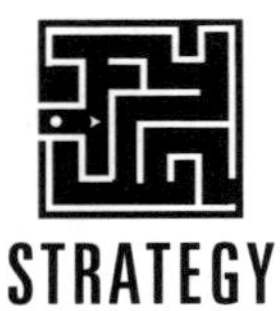

STRATEGY

Divide and Conquer. With this strategy, you separate the initial velocity vector of the projectile into horizontal and vertical components and treat these values as separate entities. "Plug and chug" these values into the appropriate kinematics equation.

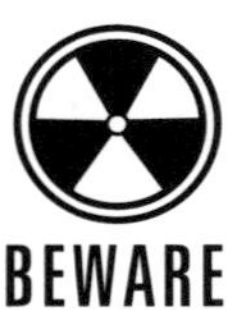

BEWARE

When calculating the total horizontal distance traveled by the projectile, simply multiply the horizontal component of the velocity (v_x) by the total time of the projectile in flight. However, when determining the total time in flight of the projectile that was fired from the ground, the answer is twice the time it takes the projectile to reach zero velocity, which occurs at the peak. Moreover, because gravity acts as a negative acceleration when the projectile is ascending, you must use $-10\ m/s^2$ for g.

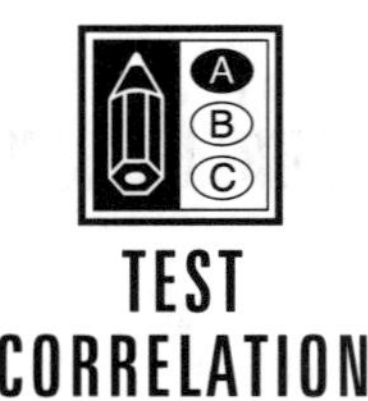

TEST CORRELATION

Projectiles are a very popular topic in the physical sciences section because they can be specifically discussed in a passage, followed by many kinematics and force questions. A passage might dramatize a rocket launch, a cannon firing, or even a ball being thrown into the air. Given the great variety of real-life applications that can be explained by projectiles, you should practice solving problems dealing with projectiles until you develop speed and accuracy.

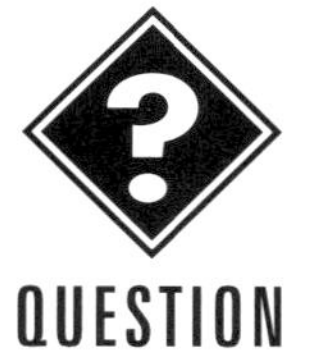

A person standing at the edge of a 200-meter cliff throws a 10-kg ball off the edge of the cliff at a 30° angle with respect to the horizontal. The ball was thrown off the cliff with an initial velocity of 20 m/s.

(a) What is the total time that the ball was in flight?

(b) How far did the ball travel horizontally?

(c) What was the maximum height that the ball attained off the ground?

The best way to solve projectile problems is to "divide and conquer" by separating the horizontal (x) and vertical (y) components of the projectile. We can begin by drawing a simple diagram of the projectile:

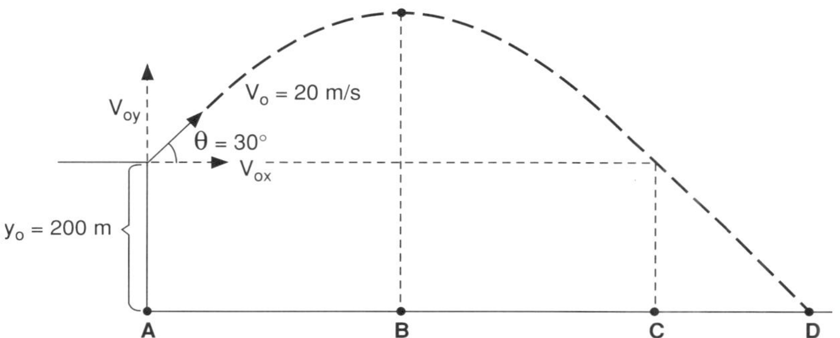

Point **A** = starting point of projectile
Point **B** = peak height of projectile
Point **C** = point where projectile returns to height of cliff
Point **D** = ending point of projectile

$V_{oy} = V_o \sin\theta = 20\ (\sin 30°) = 10$ m/s $\qquad \sin 30° = 0.5$

$V_{ox} = V_o \cos\theta = 20\ (\cos 30°) \approx 17$ m/s $\qquad \cos 30° = \frac{\sqrt{3}}{2} \approx .85$

(a) Total time in flight = time ($A \to B$) + time ($B \to C$) + time ($C \to D$), where time ($A \to B$) = time ($B \to C$)

Use the formula:

$$v = v_0 + at$$

$$v_{peak\ height} = v_{0y} - g\,[\text{time}\ (A \to B)]$$

$$0 = 10\text{ m/s} - 10\text{ m/s}^2\ [\text{time}\ (A \to B)]$$

Time ($A \to B$) = time ($B \to C$) = 1 sec

To find time (B → D), use the formula:

$$x = x_0 + v_0 t + \tfrac{1}{2} at^2$$

$$y_{\text{ground}} = y_0 - \tfrac{1}{2} gt^2$$

$$0 = 205 - (\tfrac{1}{2})(10)\,[\text{time } (C \rightarrow D)]^2$$

$$\text{Time } (B \rightarrow D) = \sqrt{41} \approx 6 \text{ sec}$$

$$\text{Therefore, time in flight} = \text{time } (A \rightarrow B) + \text{time } (B \rightarrow D)$$

$$= 1 \text{ sec} + 6 \text{ sec} = \mathbf{7\ sec}$$

(b) Because the ball was thrown at an initial velocity of 20 m/s with no component of horizontal acceleration,

$$\text{Horizontal distance traveled} = (v_{0x})\,(\text{Total time in flight})$$

$$= 17 \text{ m/s} \times 7 \text{ sec} = \mathbf{119\ m}$$

(c) Maximum height can be determined using the following formula:

$$y_{\max} = y_0 + \left| \frac{(v_{0y})^2}{2g} \right|$$

$$y_{\max} = 200 + \left| \frac{10^2}{2(-10)} \right| = \mathbf{205\ m}$$

3 FORCES AND NEWTON'S LAWS

a. Newton's First Law

An object in motion tends to stay in motion (in the absence of friction), as an object at rest tends to remain at rest.

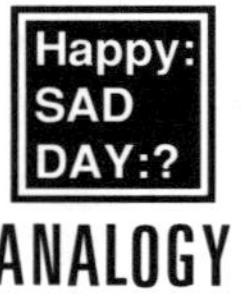

This is the law of physical inertia (as opposed to mental inertia, of which the most compelling example is the student who avoids studying).

b. Newton's Second Law

Force equals mass multiplied by acceleration:

$$F = ma$$

F = force (newtons, N, or kg·m/s^2)
m = mass (kg)
a = acceleration (m/s^2)

Another form of Newton's law follows:

$$\tau = I \times \alpha$$

τ = torque
I = moment of inertia
α = angular acceleration

Because the moment of inertia is a difficult topic for many students to grasp, think of torque as analogous to force (τ = F × radius) in the way that inertia is analogous to mass.

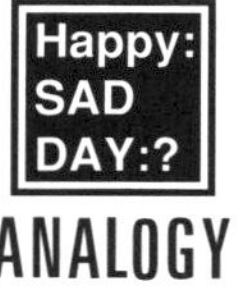

ANALOGY

c. Newton's Third Law

For every force (action), there is an equal and opposite force (reaction).

This law explains why a gun kicks back when you fire it. It kicks back due to conservation of momentum (p).

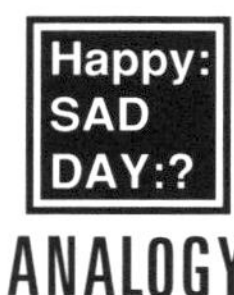

ANALOGY

d. Centripetal Force

Centripetal force is the inward force of an object as it moves in a circular path around a point. Without centripetal force, the object would move along a straight-line tangent to its circular path.

$$F = ma$$

and

$$a_c = \frac{v^2}{r}$$

Therefore,

$$F_c = m \times \frac{v^2}{r}$$

a_c = centripetal acceleration (m/s^2)
F_c = centripetal force (N)
m = mass of object (kg)
r = radius of the circular path (m)
v = velocity of object (m/s)

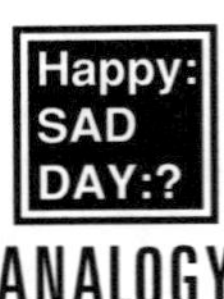

ANALOGY

This equation explains why the velocity of a car decreases rapidly as you round a turn even if your foot is on the gas pedal (unless you floor it). Turning means that you change the direction of velocity by using force, which slows down your car through friction. Similarly, if you twirl a yo-yo around your head sideways, you must pull inward on the string to keep the yo-yo orbiting at a constant speed (the way the sun keeps the earth in orbit).

e. Force of Gravity

Gravitational force is inversely related to the square of the distance between two objects, so doubling the distance between two objects would reduce gravitational force to one-fourth of its initial value.

Newton's law of gravitation states that every mass or particle in the universe is attracted to every other mass or particle by a force that is **directly** related to the masses of the objects and **inversely** related to the square of the distance between the objects. This force is called gravitational force.

$$F_g = G\frac{m_1 m_2}{r^2}$$

F_g = gravitational force (N)
m_1, m_2 = mass of each object (kg)
r = distance between the two objects (m)

G = universal gravitational constant (7×10^{-11} N·m^2/kg^2)

On the surface of the earth, m_1 is the mass of the earth (constant) and r is the radius of the earth (also fairly constant). Thus, when dealing with gravitational problems that take place on earth, the simplified form of the equation may be used:

$$F_g = mg$$

F_g = gravitational force (N)
m = mass of object (kg)
g = gravitational constant (9.8 m/s^2) = $\frac{Gm_1}{r}$

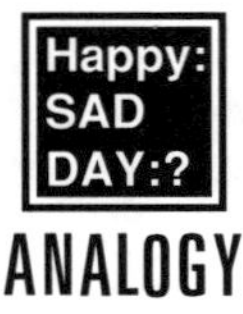

ANALOGY

Note the similarity between this equation and the equation for electricity and magnetism (F = qE), or Coulomb's law. Electricity and magnetism are difficult topics for many students to grasp; it may help to think of mass as similar to charge and force being similar to electric field strength multiplied by charge.

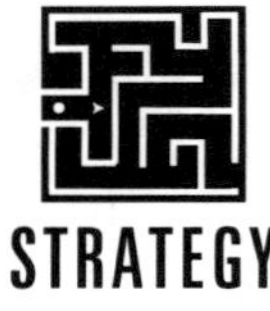
STRATEGY

When you are solving problems dealing with forces, draw a **free-body diagram** of all the forces acting on the object.

4 INCLINED PLANES

a. Forces on an Incline

On an inclined plane, the acceleration of the object going down the inclined plane is not equal to the acceleration due to gravity. Instead, you must take into account the angle of the inclined plane:

$$F = mg\sin(\theta) = ma$$
$$a = g\sin(\theta)$$

F = force on the object (N)
g = gravitational constant (9.8 m/s^2)
a = acceleration (m/s^2)
m = mass of the object (kg)
θ = angle between the inclined plane and the horizontal axis

b. Friction

Working against gravitational force is a frictional force (f) that opposes the motion of the object going down the inclined plane. The force of friction always acts directly opposite to the direction of motion.

You can see, then, why it is easier to push an object up a smooth inclined plane as opposed to lifting an object off the ground; the angle decreases the component of gravitational force opposing the plane of motion, and the smooth inclined plane has a small coefficient of friction (μ). Look at the following equation and Figure 2-1.

$$f = \mu mg\cos(\theta) = \mu F_N$$

f = frictional force (N)
m = mass of object (kg)
θ = angle between the inclined plane and the horizontal axis
μ = coefficient of friction
g = gravitational constant (9.8 m/s^2)
F_N = normal force acting on the object (N)
F_g = gravitational force acting on the object (N)

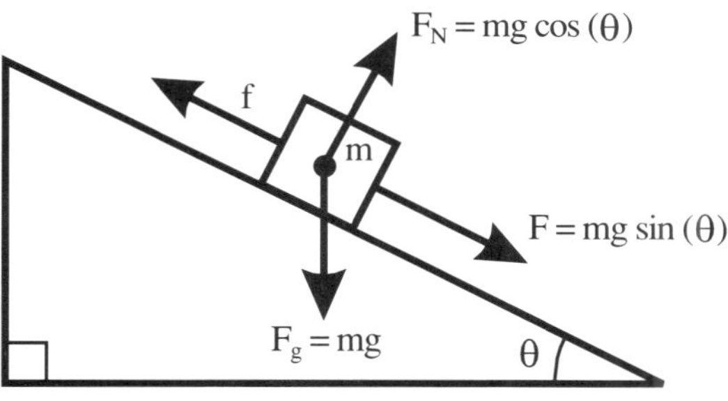

Note the forces acting on the object; for example, gravitational force, normal force, and frictional force.

Figure 2-1.
Object on an inclined plane: Free-body diagram.

5 SPRINGS, HOOKE'S LAW, AND SIMPLE HARMONIC MOTION

a. Pendulums and Springs

Pendulums and springs are two examples of systems that exhibit simple harmonic motion (Figure 2-2). A pendulum consists of a mass suspended by a string, with the upper end of the string fixed to a point. A spring system consists of a mass affixed to the end of a spring, with the upper end of the spring fixed to a point.

Note that the period of a simple pendulum does not vary with the mass of the pendulum or with the height of its swing; **the only variable that affects the period is the length of the pendulum.**

Hooke's law describes the force exerted on a mass at the end of a spring when the spring is displaced from its position of rest.

$$F = -kx$$

F = force (N)
k = spring constant (N/m)
x = displacement (m)

b. Potential Energy of a Spring

When a spring is elongated or shortened through displacement, the spring stores an elastic potential energy. Through subsequent movement, this potential energy can be converted to kinetic energy. The total energy of the spring system is:

$$E = \frac{k}{2} x^2$$

E = total energy (N·m)
k = spring constant (N/m)
x = displacement (m)

c. Period of a Simple Pendulum

The period of motion of a simple pendulum is the time it takes for the mass to undergo one full cycle of motion:

$$T = 2\pi\sqrt{\frac{l}{g}}$$

T = period of motion (s)
l = length of pendulum (m)
g = gravitational constant (9.8 m/s^2)

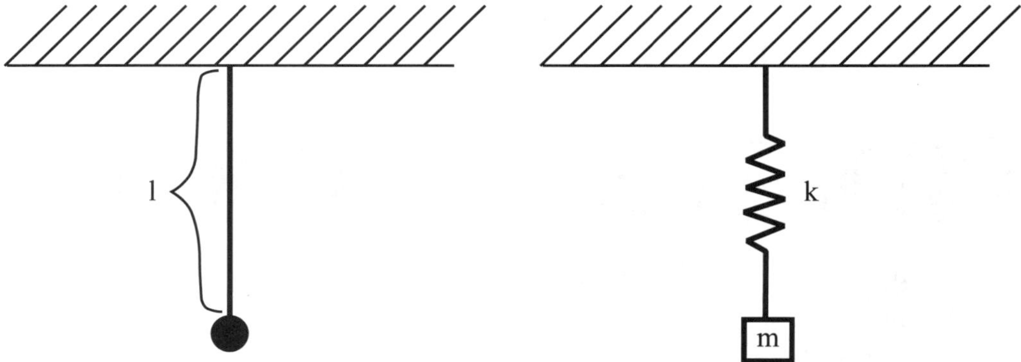

Figure 2-2.
A simple pendulum and a mass–spring system. l = Length of the pendulum string (m); m = mass of the object (kg); k = spring force constant (N/m).

d. Period of a Simple Harmonic Oscillator

The period of a simple harmonic oscillator (such as a spring system) is the time required for the spring to complete one cycle.

$$T = 2\pi\sqrt{\frac{m}{k}}$$

T = period of motion (s)
m = mass at the end of the spring (kg)
k = spring constant (N/m)

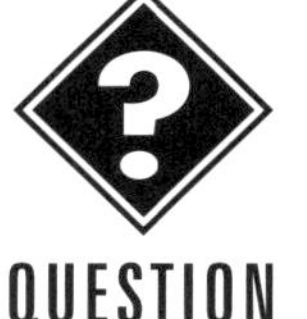

For a simple pendulum
(a) At which point does the greatest velocity occur?
(b) If the length of the string is doubled, what happens to the period of the pendulum?
(c) If the mass at the end of the pendulum is doubled, what happens to the period of the pendulum?

(a) The pendulum accelerates until it reaches its vertical orientation; therefore, its velocity is greatest when it is vertically oriented.
(b) Given that

$$T = 2\pi\sqrt{\frac{l}{g}}$$

If

$$l' = 2l, \text{ then } T' = T\sqrt{2}$$

(c) Trick question! (Yes, you will find them on the MCAT.) Notice that m (mass) is not part of the preceding equation. The period of oscillation for the pendulum does not change.

6 WORK AND ENERGY

a. Force

Strictly defined, force is what causes an object (mass) to accelerate in a particular direction. As discussed earlier, Newton's second law states that force equals mass times acceleration, or F = ma.

b. Work

is defined as the product of the force exerted on an object times the distance that the object is displaced by that force. If you hold a weight over your head, you are not doing work (although it may feel as though you are) because work is done only when a mass is moved over a certain distance by applying a force (e.g., dragging an object up an inclined plane or weight-lifting). Work is measured in newton-meters (N·m) or joules (J). Note that 1 J = 1 N·m.

$$W = F \times d$$

w = work (J)
F = force (N)
d = distance (m)

c. Kinetic energy

is the energy associated with the movement of an object.

$$KE = \frac{1}{2} mv^2$$

KE = kinetic energy (J)
m = mass (kg)
v = velocity (m/s)

d. Potential energy

is the energy that is stored in a system and can be converted into motion or work. The following equation describes the potential energy of a mass with respect to gravity.

$$PE = mgh$$

PE = potential energy (J)
g = gravitational constant (9.8 m/s^2)
m = mass (kg)
h = height (m)

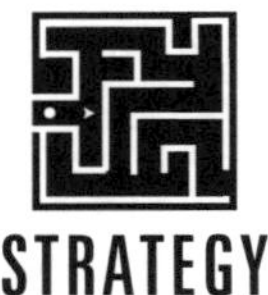
STRATEGY

By understanding the units on which physics concepts are based, you will understand and solve physics problems better than by just memorizing formulas. Try to approximate before you calculate your answer. Assume that g (gravitational acceleration) is approximately 10 m/s^2.

e. Conservation of Energy

The total energy of a kinematic/kinetic system is always constant in the absence of relativistic effects (the Einstein stuff—not on the MCAT).

$$PE + KE = \text{constant}$$

f. Power

is the rate at which work takes place on a particular object during a given unit cf time. The standard unit of power is the watt, which equals a joule/sec.

$$P = \frac{W}{t} = F \times v$$

P = power (watts)
W = work (J)
t = time (s)
F = force (N)
v = velocity (m/s)

A 10-kg object is dropped off a 20-m building. Given negligible air resistance, what is the speed of the object just before it hits the ground?

Because air resistance is negligible, assume conservation of energy. First, note two things. At the top, the object is not in motion and kinetic energy = 0 because v = 0. However, at the top, potential energy = mgh. At the bottom, potential energy = 0 because h = 0. Therefore, according to conservation of energy:

$$KE_{bottom} = PE_{top}$$

$$\tfrac{1}{2}\, mv^2 = mgh$$

$$v = \sqrt{2\,gh} = \sqrt{2 \times 10 \times 20} = 20 \text{ m/s}$$

Note that mass appears on both sides of the equation, so it cancels out.

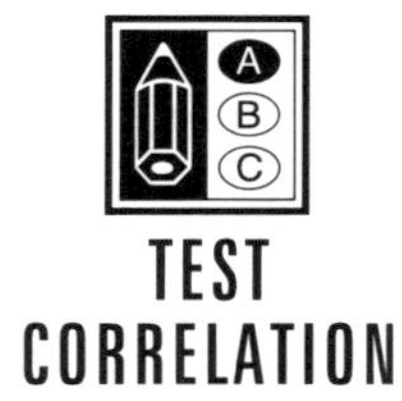

Remember that the MCAT is multiple choice. Do not waste time with excessive precision in calculations. Sometimes scanning the answers can help you decide how accurate a calculation is needed.

7 COLLISIONS: MOMENTUM AND ENERGY

a. Momentum

is the movement of an object (or mass) with a given velocity. It is measured in kg·m/s.

$$p = mv$$

p = momentum (kg·m/s)
m = mass (kg)
v = velocity (m/s)

Due to **conservation of momentum**, the final momentum of an isolated system is equal to the initial total momentum of that system.

$$\sum p_{before} = \sum p_{after}$$

In elastic collisions (e.g., when two billiard balls collide), both momentum and energy are conserved. In a perfectly elastic collision, the objects bounce off each other without any deformations in shape or structure and without any of the energy given off as heat.

In completely inelastic collisions, momentum, but not energy, is conserved. Some energy is given off as heat or is used to deform the shape or structure of the colliding objects (e.g., plasticine balls colliding and deforming).

In inelastic collisions, two bodies "stick to each other" after the collision. (You can duplicate this action by forming two balls of silly putty and making them collide.) Remember, momentum is always conserved, but energy is conserved only in a perfectly elastic collision.

b. Impulse

The impulse of a force on a mass is the change in momentum of that mass or the force applied to that mass over a given period of time.

$$i = F\Delta t = \Delta p = m\Delta v$$

i = impulse (kg·m/s)	F = force (N)
Δp = change in momentum (kg·m/s)	Δt = duration (s)
m = mass of object (kg)	Δv = change in velocity (m/s)

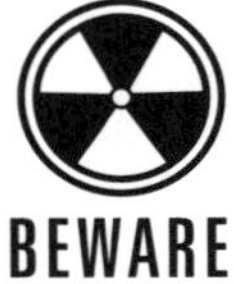

Remember that velocity and momentum are both vectors that have both a speed and a directional component. Therefore, always assign a specific direction as positive and the opposite direction as negative.

Two balls hit each other in a head-on collision. Before the collision, ball A, which has a mass of 2 kg, was moving north at a speed of 5 m/s, whereas ball B, which weighs 4 kg, was moving south at 3 m/s. After the collision, ball B is moving north at 1 m/s.

(a) What are the speed and direction of ball A after the collision?

(b) Is this collision elastic or inelastic?

In these types of problems, take into account the direction in which the balls are moving. You can arbitrarily decide that a particle traveling north has a positive velocity whereas a particle traveling south has a negative velocity.

(a) Conservation of momentum

$$\sum mv_{before} = \sum mv_{after}$$

$$(2\text{ kg})(+5\text{ m/s}) + (4\text{ kg})(-3\text{ m/s}) = (2\text{ kg})(x\text{ m/s}) + (4\text{ kg})(+1\text{ m/s})$$

$$-2 = 2x + 4$$

$$x = -3\text{ m/s}$$

Therefore, after the collision, ball A is moving south at **3 m/s.**

(b) To determine whether the collision is elastic, you need to know whether energy has been conserved:

$$\sum \frac{mv^2}{2}_{before} = ?\ \sum \frac{mv^2}{2}_{after}$$

$$(2\text{ kg})(5\text{ m/s})^2 + (4\text{ kg})(-3\text{ m/s})^2 = ?\ (2\text{ kg})(-3\text{ m/s})^2 + (4\text{ kg})(+1\text{ m/s})^2$$

$$86 \neq 22.$$

Energy is not conserved; therefore, this was an **inelastic** collision.

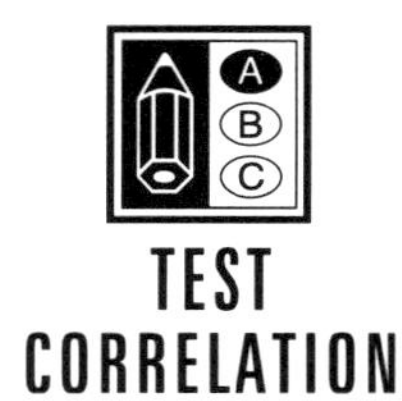

TEST CORRELATION

Momentum is frequently tested through hypothetical situations with billiard balls and collisions. Understanding of impulse is frequently tested on the MCAT in passages that involve car accidents. Because there are many motor vehicle accidents each year, collisions are a “trendy” topic that can be expected to appear on the MCAT.

8 TORQUE AND EQUILIBRIUM

a. Torque

is the tendency of a force to rotate an object about an axis. Torque (τ) is measured in N·m. Notice that the units are the same as those used for energy, but torque and energy are not the same.

$$\tau = F \times r$$

τ = torque (N·m)
F = force (N)
r = radius (m)

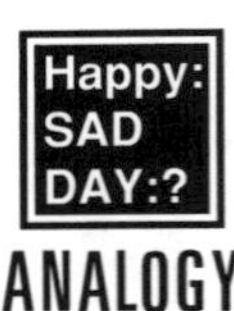

ANALOGY

This equation explains why a larger crowbar can pry things open more easily than its smaller counterpart can because the larger one (greater r) has more torque for a given force.

b. Equilibrium

In this state, the following is true:

$$\sum F = 0$$

$$\sum \tau = 0$$

QUESTION

A 2-kg uniform meter stick has a fulcrum at the 40-cm mark. A 5-kg mass rests on the 10-cm mark. A 3-kg mass rests on the 60-cm mark.

Where must a 4-kg mass rest to achieve equilibrium?

ANSWER

To solve this problem, draw the picture and **assign distances relative to the position of the fulcrum.** Remember that a uniform mass has its center of mass at its center (i.e., the meter stick acts as a mass that rests at the 50-cm mark).

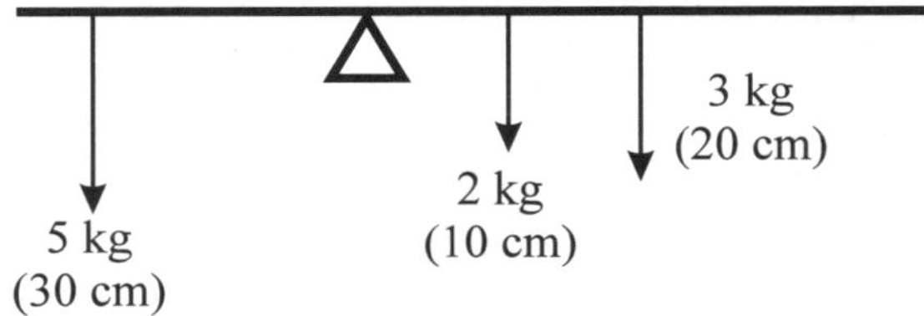

From this picture, you can set up your equation. It doesn't matter on which side you put your unknown 4-kg mass. If you put the mass on the wrong side, your answer (distance) is simply a negative number instead of a positive number.

Equilibrium

$$\sum \tau_{counterclockwise} = \sum \tau_{clockwise}$$

$$(5 \text{ kg})(30 \text{ cm}) + (4 \text{ kg})(x \text{ cm}) = (2 \text{ kg})(10 \text{ cm}) + (3 \text{ kg})(20 \text{ cm})$$

$$150 + 4x = 80$$

$$x = -17.5 \text{ cm}$$

Therefore, the 4-kg object should be 17.5 cm to the **right** of the fulcrum.

$$\text{Position of the mass} = \text{Fulcrum} + \text{Distance from the fulcrum}$$

$$= 40 \text{ cm} + 17.5 \text{ cm} = \mathbf{57.5\ cm}$$

9 SOUND AND LIGHT

a. Wavelength

is the distance required to complete one full cycle of a wave.

b. Frequency

is the rate at which cycles occur, or the number of cycles per unit of time. Frequency is measured in hertz (Hz = cycles per second).

Sound and light have constant velocities under constant conditions. Sound and light waves with high frequencies have short wavelengths and high energies. Sound and light waves with low frequencies have longer wavelengths and lower energies.

$$v = f \cdot \lambda$$

v = velocity (m/s)
f = frequency (Hz)
λ = wavelength (m)

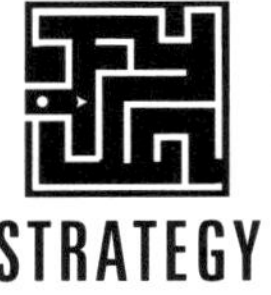

Visible light waves usually have wavelengths that are hundreds of nanometers (nm $= 10^{-9}$ m). Sound waves typically have wavelengths of several meters. Knowing these facts may help you eliminate bogus answer choices that appear on the MCAT.

c. Sound Intensity

The intensity of a sound wave is the rate at which the energy flows through a given area, or the power of the sound wave per unit area. Sound intensity is determined by the amplitude of the sound wave. Volume is often measured in decibels (dB).

Because sound intensity is inversely proportional to the square of the distance from the source, decreasing the distance from the source by one-half increases the intensity of the sound fourfold.

$$V = 10 \log \left(\frac{I}{I_0}\right) \qquad \Delta V = 10 \log \frac{I_{new}}{I_{old}}$$

V = volume of sound (dB)
I = intensity of the sound at a given point (W/m^2)
I_0 = the threshold of hearing (10^{-12} W/m^2)

I_{new} = new sound intensity (W/m^2)
I_{old} = original sound intensity (W/m^2)

A person turns up the radio from 20 dB to 40 dB. By how many fold has the intensity of the sound increased?

ANSWER

Using the preceding equation:

$$\Delta V = 10 \log \left(\frac{I_{new}}{I_{old}}\right)$$

$$40 - 20 = 10 \log \left(\frac{I_{new}}{I_{old}}\right)$$

$$2 = \log \left(\frac{I_{new}}{I_{old}}\right)$$

$$\frac{I_{new}}{I_{old}} = 100\text{-fold}$$

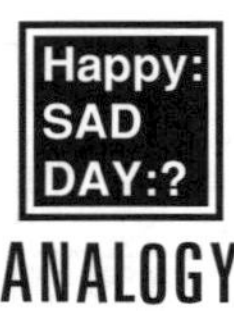

ANALOGY

In chemistry, pH also works on a log scale. Therefore, you should understand the 100-fold difference in hydrogen ion concentration between a pH 2 and a pH 4 solution.

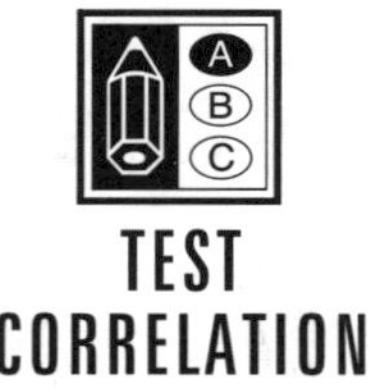

TEST CORRELATION

Waves are basic to many physics topics (e.g., sound, light, and kinematics ; therefore, questions involving the formula v = fλ are popular on the MCAT. In fact, this equation appears on the MCAT so often that we have dubbed v = fλ "MCAT's favorite formula." You should be able to link concepts of waves to sound, light, and kinematics. Expect to use the formula v = fλ and to see at least one question (maybe even a whole passage) involving waves.

QUESTION

A laser that emits a 500-nm beam of light passes from air (n = 1) through a tank of water (n = 1.33) that has a diameter of 25 m.

(a) What is the velocity of the light wave as it passes through the tank of water?

(b) What is the frequency of the light wave?

(c) By what percentage is the original speed of the light wave reduced as it passes from air to water?

(d) How long does it take the light wave to traverse the tank of water?

ANSWER

(a) $v_{H_2O} = c/n$

$v_{H_2O} = 3 \times 10^8/1.33 \approx 2.25 \times 10^8$ m/s

(b) $v = f\lambda_{air}$

$f = v_{air}/\lambda_{air} = 3 \times 10^8/500 \times 10^{-9} = 6 \times 10^{14}$ Hz

(c) $\Delta v = \dfrac{n_{air}}{n_{H_2O}} = \dfrac{1}{1.33} = 0.75 \qquad 1 - 0.75 = 0.25$

Therefore, the speed of the wave decreased by **25%.**

(d) $x = v_0 t$

$25 = 2.25 \times 10^8\,(t)$

$t = \dfrac{25}{2.25 \times 10^8} \approx 1 \times 10^{-7}$ sec

10 OPTICS

a. Reflection

Reflection occurs when light rays traveling in a given medium encounter a second medium and travel back from the boundary between the two media. The angle of the reflected ray always equals the angle of the incident ray.

$$\theta_{incident} = \theta_{reflected}$$

b. Refraction

When light rays traveling in a given medium encounter a second medium and travel into it, they bend (refract) at the boundary between the two media. *Snell's law* concerns the angle of the refracted ray.

Snell's law. Light changes its direction of propagation at an interface between two media (e.g., air and glass, as in Figure 2-3). The angle of refraction of a beam of light (θ_r) depends on its angle of incidence (θ_i) at this surface, as follows:

$$n_r \sin(\theta_r) = n_i \sin(\theta_i)$$

n_r, n_i = indices of refraction of the refractive and incident media

θ_r, θ_i = angle of the refracted and incident rays with respect to a plane **perpendicular to the reflecting surface** (see Figure 2-3).

HIGH-YIELD FACTS

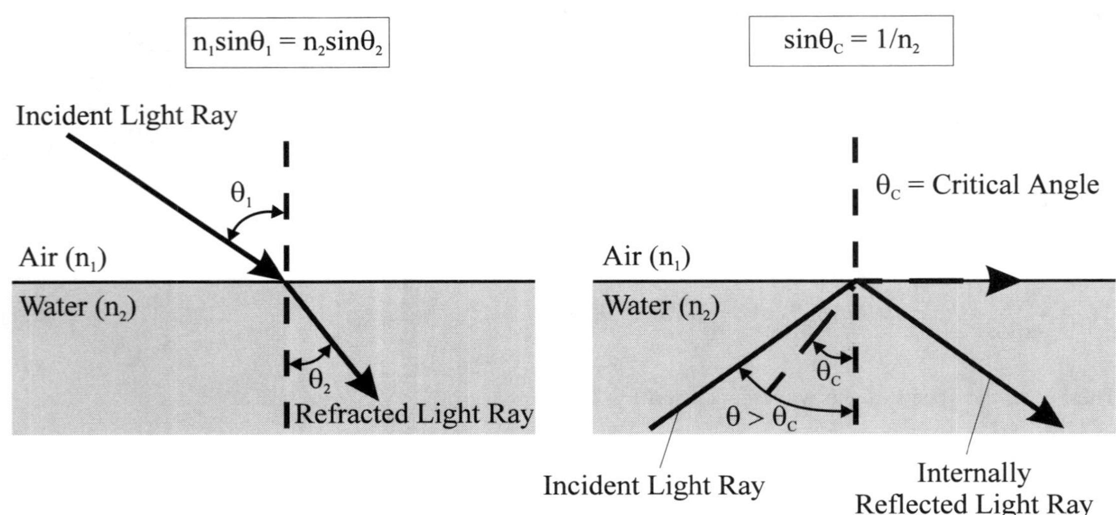

Figure 2-3.
Refraction and reflection.

Critical angle is the angle of incidence (θ_i) for which the angle of refraction (θ_r) is 90°.

$$\sin(\theta_{critical}) = \frac{n_r}{n_i}$$

$\theta_{critical}$ = critical angle
n_r, n_i = indices of refraction of the refractive and incident media

A critical angle exists only when light is traveling from a more optically dense medium to a less optically dense medium. If the angle of incidence is higher than the critical angle, no refraction occurs. The ray of light instead experiences total internal reflection, which is how diamonds sparkle.

You should be aware of how the properties of light waves change when light passes into a more dense medium (e.g., $n_{glass} = 1.5$) from a less dense medium (e.g., $n_{air} = 1$). When light waves pass into a medium with a higher index of refraction (i.e., a more dense medium):

1. velocity decreases because $n = c/v$ (velocity is inversely proportional to the index of refraction).
2. frequency of the wave remains unchanged.
3. the energy of the wave remains unchanged, and this wave energy is directly proportional to the wave frequency $E = hf = hc/\lambda$.
4. wavelength decreases (i.e., **"blue shift"** occurs because velocity decreases and frequency remains unchanged, via $v = f\lambda$).
5. the angle of the ray of light relative to the normal is smaller (the beam bends back toward the normal as in the preceding diagram, per Snell's law).

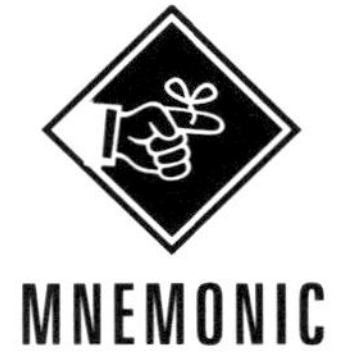
MNEMONIC

Therefore, when a light wave passes from a less dense to a more dense medium, it gets **slower and bluer.**

When the homework you're doing gets more and more dense, you get the "blues" and are slow to get things done.

c. Lensmaker's Equation

If you know the distance of an object (d_o) from a lens of known focal length (f), the following equation lets you calculate the position (d_i) of the image formed from the lens:

$$\frac{1}{f} = \frac{1}{d_o} + \frac{1}{d_i} = \frac{2}{r}$$

f = focal length of lens (m)
d_i = distance of the image from the lens (m)
d_o = distance of the object from the lens (m)
r = radius of curvature of the lens (m)

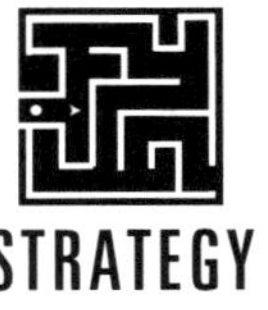
STRATEGY

For both a lens and a mirror, a positive image distance d_i is characteristic of a real image (the image formed is composed of light that is really present). A negative d_i represents a virtual image (the image observed is **not** formed from real light). A positive focal-length value occurs only in a converging lens or mirror, whereas a negative focal length is consistent with a diverging lens or mirror (Figure 2-4). For a diverging lens, the image is always virtual, erect, and smaller (Table 2-1). Lenses and mirrors bend light rays in opposite ways. A convex lens and a concave mirror are both converging ($f > 0$), whereas a concave lens and a convex mirror are both diverging ($f < 0$).

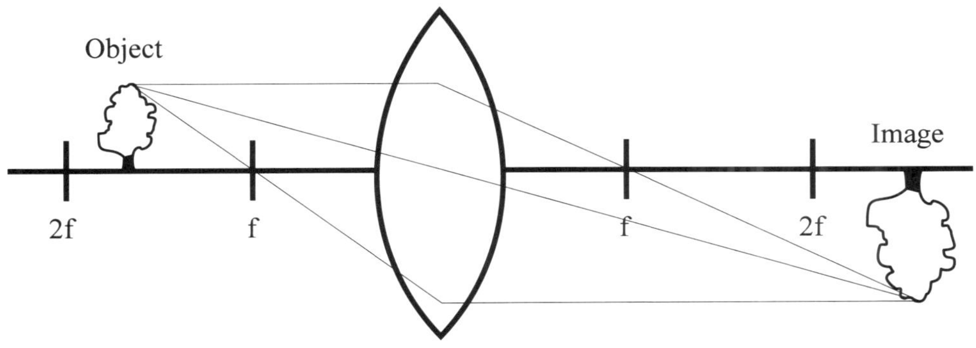

An object placed between the focal distance and the radius of curvature (2f) of a converging lens will form a real image that is inverted and larger than the object.

Figure 2-4.
A converging lens.

TABLE 2-1. Image using converging and diverging lenses

Condition	Converging Lens Image	Diverging Lens Image
$d_o < f$	Virtual, erect, larger	Virtual, erect, smaller
$f < d_o < 2f$	Real, inverted, larger	Virtual, erect, smaller
$d_o = 2f$	Real, inverted, same size	Virtual, erect, smaller
$d_o > 2f$	Real, inverted, smaller	Virtual, erect, smaller

1. **Magnification.** The relative height of an image compared to its object is the same as the ratio of their distances from the lens:

$$M = \frac{-d_i}{d_o} = \frac{h_i}{h_o}$$

M = magnification ratio
d_i = distance of image (m)
d_o = distance of object (always positive, m)
h_i = height of image (m)
h_o = height of object (m)

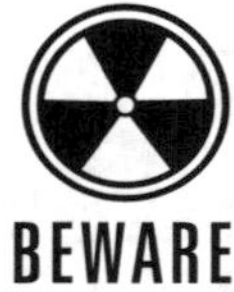
BEWARE

If the magnification ratio (M) is positive, the image is erect. If M is negative, the image is inverted.

2. **Diopter** is a unit of refractory power in which the focal distance of the lens is in meters. Diopters (not focal lengths) are additive.

$$D = \frac{1}{f}$$

D = diopter (m^{-1})
f = focal length (m)

For example, a converging lens with a focal length of +20 cm (0.2 m) is a +5 diopter lens:

$$+5 \text{ diopters} = \frac{1}{0.2 \text{ m}}$$

11 SOUND

Sound must travel through a medium; it does **not** travel in a vacuum. Therefore, one cannot hear an explosion in outer space (one of the many flaws in movies about outer space).

Sound is transmitted by the vibration of particles within the medium (which is why your room shakes if you crank up the bass on your stereo). The higher the density of the

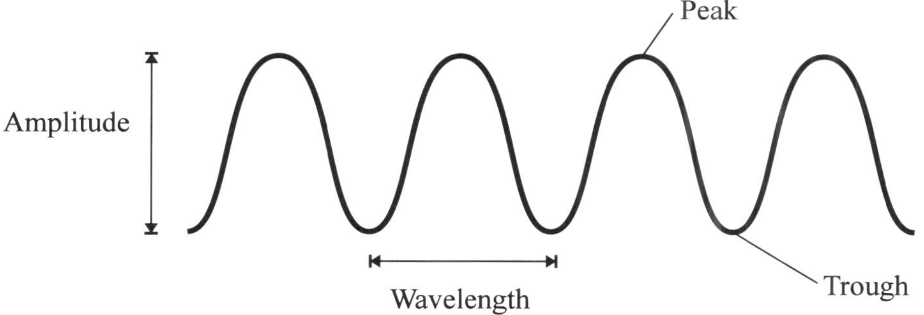

Figure 2-5. A sound wave.

medium, the greater the speed of sound. Pitch is determined by, and proportional to, the frequency of the sound wave. Intensity is determined by the amplitude of the sound wave (Figure 2-5).

a. Beats and Beat Frequency

The superposition of two waves of slightly different wavelengths and frequencies gives rise to beats. Specific beats are observed as oscillations of the amplitude of the entire pattern. The beat frequency is:

$$f_{beat} = |f_1 - f_2|$$

f_{beat} = beat frequency (Hz)
f_1, f_2 = frequencies of overlapping waves (Hz)

QUESTION

When two sounds are different, one 330 Hz and the other 320 Hz, what is the beat frequency?

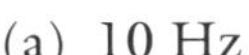
(a) 10 Hz

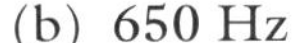
(b) 650 Hz

(c) 5 Hz

(d) 20 Hz

(e) 0 Hz

ANSWER

The correct answer is (a). Recall that:

$$\begin{aligned} f_{beat} &= |f_1 - f_2| \\ &= |\,330\text{ Hz} - 320\text{ Hz}\,| = 10\text{ Hz} \end{aligned}$$

QUESTION

If a piano key is hit simultaneously with a 400-Hz note on a nearby xylophone, a beat with a frequency of 15 Hz is produced. What is the frequency of the piano key?

I. 385 Hz

II. 400 Hz

III. 415 Hz

(a) I only

(b) II only

(c) III only

(d) I and III only

(e) Cannot be determined from information given

ANSWER

The correct answer is (d). Plugging the answers into the preceding equation shows that I and III would produce a beat with a frequency of 15 Hz, whereas II would not produce a beat at all.

b. Doppler Effect

The Doppler effect describes the change in sound frequency that results from motion of the source relative to a sound detector.

$$f' = f\,\frac{v \pm v_d}{v \mp v_s}$$

f' = new frequency (Hz)

f = original frequency (Hz)

v_s = velocity of sound source (m/s)

v_d = velocity of sound detector (m/s)

QUESTION

If a car is accelerating as it comes toward you with its horn honking, does the sound of the horn:

(a) increase in pitch

(b) decrease in pitch

(c) decrease in volume

(d) increase in volume

(e) increase in pitch and volume

ANSWER

The correct answer is (e). You know from experience that a horn sounds louder when a car approaches at rapid speed (because intensity is inversely proportional to the square of the distance from the source). The pitch of the horn increases to a higher note, just as pitch increases when you hear a police car blaring its siren as it moves toward you. As the car (or police car) moves past you, the pitch decreases rapidly—the Doppler effect.

Standing waves and closed or open nodes. The amplitude of the wave at the closed end of a pipe, for a standing wave, is always zero (node). The amplitude of a standing wave at the open end of a pipe is always maximal (antinode). When a pipe is closed at one end, the standing wave created has a maximum wavelength of four times the length of the pipe. A pipe with both ends open or closed can support a standing wave whose maximal wavelength is two times the length of the pipe (Figure 2-6).

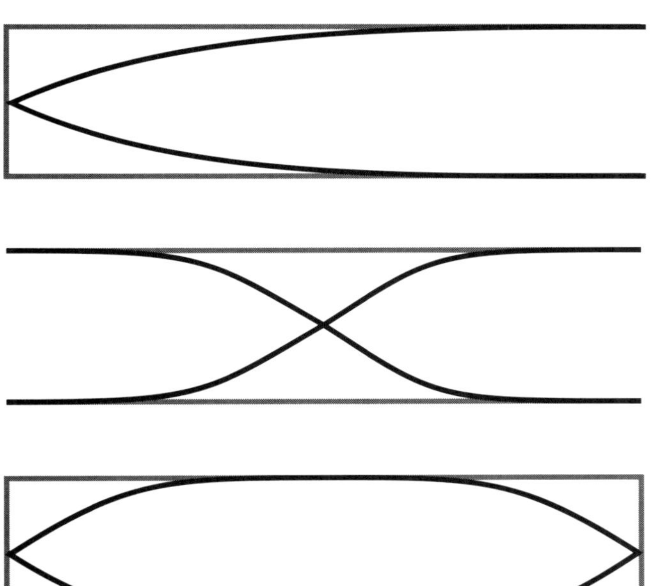

Pipe closed at one end:

$$\text{wavelength} = \frac{4(l)}{n}$$

where n = 1, 3, 5, 7, ...

Pipe with both ends closed or open:

$$\text{wavelength} = \frac{2(l)}{n}$$

where n = 1, 2, 3, 4, ...

Figure 2-6.
Standing waves in pipes.

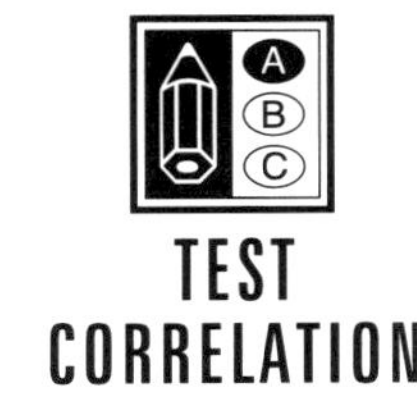

TEST CORRELATION

Doppler echocardiography (an imaging technique akin to sonar that uses ultrasound waves to view heart structures) is a recent advance in medical technology. The writers of the MCAT may pose questions about the Doppler effect to be sure that you understand this emerging technology.

12 FLUIDS AND HEAT TRANSFER

a. Fluid Flow

The two types of fluid flow are laminar and turbulent.

1. **Laminar flow** occurs when a liquid flows at a steady rate, and all of the flow is generally in one direction.
2. **Turbulent flow** occurs when the liquid moves in all directions and there is a loss of energy caused by the movement. In this instance, some of the flow equations, mainly Bernoulli's equation, do not apply.

Laminar flow occurs in the middle of a pipe or blood vessel, whereas turbulent flow occurs more often at the periphery of a pipe or a blood vessel.

b. Pressure Changes

1. **Pressure** is force per unit area:

$$P = \frac{F}{A}$$

P = pressure (pascals [Pa = N/m^2])
F = force (newtons, N)
A = area (m^2)

A pressure difference can be described in terms of the fluid flow rate and the resistance to flow:

$$\Delta P = \Phi \cdot R$$

ΔP = change in pressure
Φ = flow
R = resistance

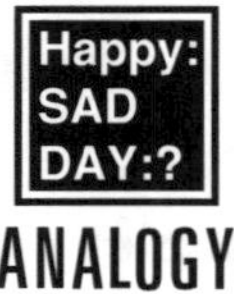

ANALOGY

You must understand the concept of resistance. It applies not only to pressure, but also to circuits, which you can see in Ohm's law, where V = IR (see Part II D 14 a). Voltage is analogous to pressure gradient; current is analogous to flow.

2. **Poiseuille's law** describes the resistance to flow of a fluid through a pipe. It states that resistance (R) is directly proportional to the viscosity (η) of the fluid and inversely proportional to the fourth power of the radius (r) of the tube or vessel of length (L) in which it flows.

$$R = \frac{8\eta L}{r^4}$$

R = resistance η = viscosity
L = length r = radius

3. **Continuity Equation.** For steady flow, which means that the same amount of fluid that enters an area will leave that area, the speed of flow along a small group of associated streamlines decreases with increasing cross-sectional area.

Fluid velocity is inversely proportional to the cross-sectional area of the pipe or blood vessel.

$$A_1 v_1 = A_2 v_2$$

A_1, A_2 = cross-sectional area of the entering and leaving streamline bundle
v_1, v_2 = flow velocity in the entering and exiting streamline bundle

Fluid dynamics are a trendy MCAT topic because they apply to blood circulation and organ perfusion.

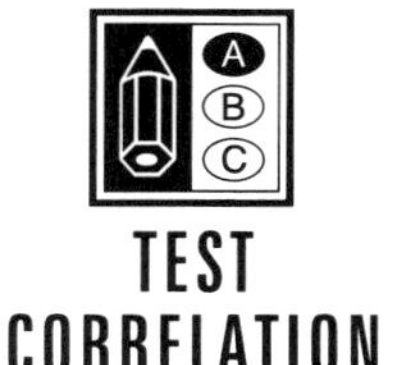

TEST CORRELATION

4. **Bernoulli's Equation.** For a given streamline, the sum of the pressure, the potential energy density, and the kinetic energy density is a constant.

$$P + \rho g h + \frac{1}{2}\rho v^2 = \text{constant}$$

P = pressure
ρ = density
g = gravitational constant
h = height
v = flow velocity

Clearly, then, if an element of fluid increases its height along a stream, either its velocity or pressure must decrease.

The diameter of the brand new water gun for your sprinkler is one-third the diameter of the hose. If water flows through the hose at 10 m/s, how rapidly does the water flow out of the water gun?

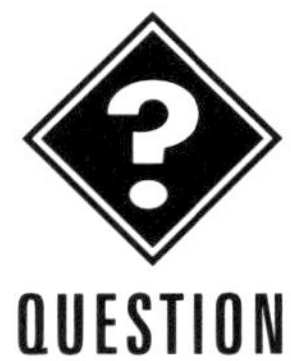

QUESTION

The cross-sectional area of the hose is nine times the area of the water gun (the area of a circle is proportional to the square of the radius). According to the continuity equation:

$$A_{hose} \times v_{hose} = A_{gun} \times v_{gun}$$

Because $A_{\text{hose}} = 9A_{\text{gun}}$, $9A_{\text{gun}} \times v_{\text{hose}} = A_{\text{gun}} \times v_{\text{gun}}$; therefore, $v_{\text{gun}} = 9 \times v_{\text{hose}}$. Hence, the velocity of the water flowing out of the water gun is 9 (10 m/s) = 90 m/s.

ANSWER

QUESTION

An atherosclerotic plaque occludes a blood vessel and decreases the radius of the vessel to half its original size. How much would pressure need to increase to maintain the same amount of blood flow in the vessel?

ANSWER

Poiseuille's law shows that resistance is inversely proportional to r^4.

$$\Delta P = FR = F\frac{8\eta L}{r^4}$$

By reducing r to its original size, R and thus ΔP increase by 2^4 (i.e., by 16). The same amount of flow would thus require 16 times the original pressure, a situation that could easily lead to a heart attack or stroke.

c. Heat Transfer

The three mechanisms of heat transfer are conduction, convection, and radiation.

1. **Conduction.** Heat transfer occurs through the direct contact of two objects.
2. **Convection.** Heat transfer occurs through the random motion of particles in the heated material.
3. **Radiation.** Heat transfer occurs through the emission of electromagnetic waves.

13 ELECTROSTATICS AND ELECTROMAGNETISM

a. Electric Fields

A gravitational field is associated with mass, and an electric field is associated with charge. An electric field (E) exerts a force on a charged particle (q) as follows:

$$F = qE$$

F = force (N)
q = charge (coulombs)
E = electric field strength (volts/m, V/m)

b. Voltage

Voltage is the potential energy per unit charge. The voltage difference is often defined operationally as the work (W) necessary to move a charge (q) from one position to another.

$$V = \frac{W}{q}$$

Many people find electromagnetism more challenging than mechanics; using the analogies that follow, you can tackle electrostatics and electromagnetism in the same way that you solve kinematics equations.

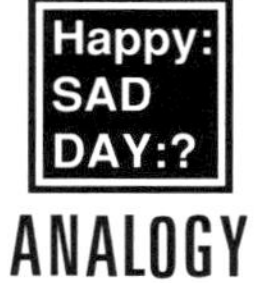

ANALOGY

Think of charge (q) as analogous to mass (m), and an electric field (E) as analogous to the acceleration (a). Then, the equation $F = qE$ is analogous to $F = ma$, and the equation $F = kq_1q_2/r^2$ is analogous to $F = Gm_1m_2/r^2$.

14 ELECTRICITY, CIRCUITS, RESISTANCE, AND CAPACITANCE

a. Ohm's Law

The electrical potential between two points depends on the current and the resistance to current flow:

$$V = IR$$

V = voltage (volts, V)
I = current (amperes, amp)
R = resistance (ohms, Ω)

b. Power

As discussed in the kinematics section, power is the work expended per unit time (power = work/time). The electrical expression for power is:

$$P = IV = I^2R = \frac{V^2}{R}$$

P = power (watts, W)
V = voltage (volts, V)
I = current (amperes, amp)
R = resistance (ohms, Ω)

c. Resistance

The resistance to current flow increases with wire length and decreases with wire cross-sectional area.

$$R = \frac{\rho_0 L}{A}$$

R = resistance (ohms, Ω)
L = wire length (m)
ρ_0 = resistivity (property of material of the wire)
A = cross-sectional area of the wire (m^2)

d. Resistance of a Circuit

Deriving an equivalent resistance of a circuit to represent complex clusters of resistors is a good first step in tackling a circuit problem.

1. **Resistors in series.** In this situation, several resistors are strewn along a single path of wire. The resistance (R_{eq}) of a set of resistors in series is the sum of the component resistors:

$$R_{eq} = R_1 + R_2 + R_3$$

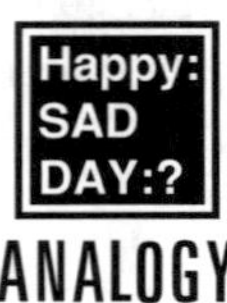

ANALOGY

This example of resistance is the famous scenario of the cheap Christmas lights. The current must flow through all of the resistors (lights), so shutting off one light opens the entire circuit and causes all the lights to go off.

2. **Resistors in parallel.** In this situation, several parallel paths of wire, each with its own resistor, travel downstream and later merge. The equivalent resistance (R_{eq}) of a set of resistors aligned in parallel is determined by:

$$\frac{1}{R_{eq}} = \frac{1}{R_1} + \frac{1}{R_2} + \frac{1}{R_3}$$

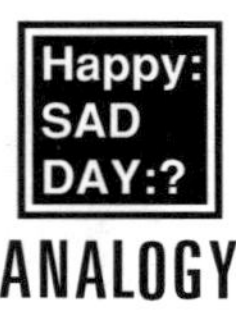

ANALOGY

When Christmas lights are arranged in parallel and you shut off one light, the current through each bulb stays the same, but the total current decreases. Thus, the remaining lights are unaffected.

e. Capacitance

Two plates of area (A) and separation distance (d) define a capacitor. Capacitance can be thought of as a measure of the storage of charge per volt. **Dielectrics,** which increase ε_0 relative to air, decrease the effective distance (d) between the plates of the capacitor, thereby causing:

- Increase of capacitance
- Decrease of voltage across the capacitor

$$C = \varepsilon_0 \frac{A}{d}$$

C = capacitance (farads, F)
A = plate area
ε_0 = dielectric constant of the medium between the two plates
d = distance separating the plates

The capacitance is related to the charge (q) and the voltage (V) of a circuit as follows:

$$q = CV$$

q = charge (coulombs)
C = capacitance
V = voltage

f. Voltage Across a Capacitor

The voltage (V) across a capacitor equals the electric field (E) across the capacitor times the distance (d) between the plates:

$$V = Ed$$

g. Capacitance of a Circuit

Like equivalent resistance, equivalent capacitance is a useful concept.

1. **Capacitors in series.** The equivalent capacitance of a set of capacitors placed in series along a single path of wire is calculated as follows:

$$\frac{1}{C_{eq}} = \frac{1}{C_1} + \frac{1}{C_2} + \frac{1}{C_3}$$

2. **Capacitors in parallel.** The equivalent capacitance derived for capacitors placed on parallel paths in a circuit is the sum of the contributing capacitances.

$$C_{eq} = C_1 + C_2 + C_3$$

Capacitors **in series** have the **same charge** (q); capacitors in **parallel** have the **same voltage** (V).

QUESTION

What is the resistance of a 100-watt lightbulb that is plugged into a 120-volt DC circuit?

ANSWER

$$P = \frac{V^2}{R}$$

P = power (watts, W)
V = voltage (volts, V)
R = resistance (ohms, Ω)

Rearranging the equation:

$$R = \frac{V^2}{P} = \frac{120^2}{100} = 144\ \Omega$$

15 RIGHT-HAND RULE

The magnitude and direction of the magnetic force (F) on a wire of length (L) depend on the magnitude and direction of the magnetic field (B) and the length of the wire:

$$F = ILB \sin(\theta)$$

F = force (N)
I = current (amp)
L = length of wire (m)
B = strength of the magnetic field (gauss)
θ = angle between vector B and wire

The right-hand rule has many versions. You may have learned a different one. Nevertheless, you should use the version given here, so you won't be confused.

The direction of the force, current, or magnetic field can be predicted if you know the other two directions and use the right-hand rule.

- Place your index finger in the direction of motion of a positively charged particle (i.e., point it in the opposite direction if the particle is an electron).
- Place digits 3–5 in the direction of the magnetic field.
- Your thumb points in the direction of the force.

QUESTION

If an electron particle is traveling to the right as it enters a magnetic field that is moving as shown, what is the direction of the force that acts on the electron when it enters the magnetic field?

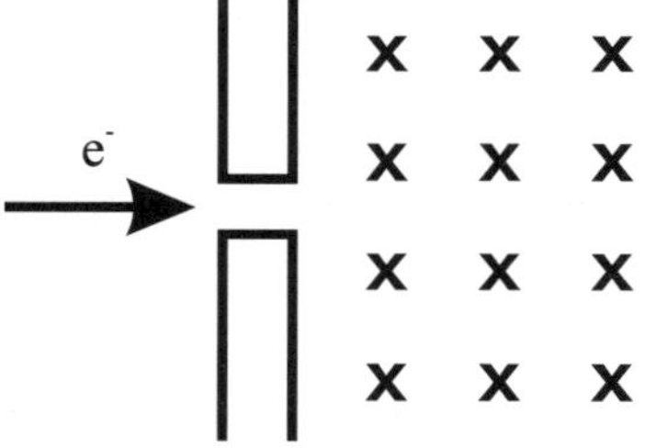

ANSWER

Using the right-hand rule, the index finger points to the left because this example deals with an electron (negative charge). Other fingers are pointing into the page. Your thumb (i.e., the force) should be pointing **down**.

16 ELECTROMAGNETIC ENERGY

Electromagnetic waves (with constant speed $c = 3 \times 10^8$ m/s) include a vast range of frequencies, from radio waves at the lower end to gamma rays at the higher end of the spectrum (Figure 2-7). The energy of these waves is directly proportional to their frequency (f) and inversely proportional to their wavelength (λ):

$$E = hf = h\frac{c}{\lambda}$$

E = energy of light (J)
f = frequency (Hz)
λ = wavelength of light (m)

h = Planck's constant
c = speed of light (m/s)

Remember

$$E = mc^2$$

E = energy
m = mass
c = speed of light

Based on the preceding equations, the higher the frequency is, the higher the energy; so gamma rays can be more dangerous to human tissue than x-rays.

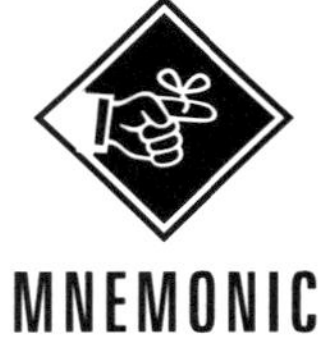
MNEMONIC

In the visible spectrum, **ROY G. BIV** describes the order of colors from **low to high frequency,** and from **long to short wavelengths.**

R Red
O Orange
Y Yellow
G Green
B Blue
I Indigo
V Violet

AM Radio waves	FM, TV	Microwaves	Infrared	Visible	Ultraviolet	X-rays	Gamma Rays	
< 10^9 Hz	10^9 Hz	10^{11} Hz	10^{14} Hz		10^{17} Hz	10^{19} Hz	> 10^{19} Hz	⇦ Frequency (Hz)

Red	Orange	Yellow	Green	Blue	Violet	
700-630λ	630-590λ	590-560λ	560-480λ	480-440λ	440-400λ	⇦ Wavelength (nm)

Figure 2-7.
The electromagnetic spectrum.

17 NUCLEAR PHYSICS

a. Atomic number

is the number of protons in the nucleus of an atom, which equals the number of electrons in a neutral element (Table 2-2).

TABLE 2-2. Subatomic particles

Particle	Alternate Name	Symbol	Mass Number	Atomic Number
Alpha	Helium nucleus	α	4	2
Beta	Electron	β	0	−1
Gamma		γ	0	0
Neutron		n	1	0
Positron		β^+	0	1

b. Mass number

is the total number of protons and neutrons in the nucleus of an atom.

c. Isotopes

are two atoms with the same atomic number but different mass numbers; they differ in the number of neutrons in the nucleus.

d. Atomic Mass

A "weighted average" of the mass numbers for the different isotopes of a particular element is the average mass of an atom of a particular element and is equal to the number of grams in a mole of that element.

^{235}U (atomic number 92) undergoes spontaneous radioactive decay after colliding with a neutron. It emits four alpha particles, two beta particles, and three gamma particles. What atom is formed?

You know that mass is conserved in all reactions, so all you have to do is write out the reaction, as follows:

$$^{235}_{92}U + {}^{1}_{0}n \rightarrow {}^{16}_{8}\alpha_4 + {}^{0}_{-2}\beta_2 + {}^{0}_{0}\gamma_3 + {}^{a}_{b}X$$

Adding up the top and bottom numbers results in two simple equations:

$$236 = 16 + \text{mass number } (a)$$

$$92 = 6 + \text{atomic number } (b)$$

Mass number = 220
Atomic number = 86

By looking at the periodic table, you see that radon (Rn) has an atomic number of 86. (The periodic table is included in the MCAT question booklet.) Therefore, the answer is ^{220}Rn.

18 RADIOACTIVE DECAY AND HALF-LIFE

Half-life is the time required for half the particles of a given substance to decay radioactively. For radioactive decay, the fraction of particles left (A/A_0) at time (t) is:

$$\frac{A}{A_0} = \left(\frac{1}{2}\right)^{t/t_{1/2}}$$

A = number of particles A_0 = initial number of particles
$t_{1/2}$ = half-life t = time

When time (t) equals the half-life ($t_{1/2}$), $A/A_0 = 1/2$.

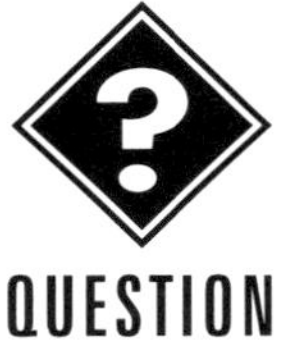

If radioactive substance X has a half-life of 3 hours, approximately how long will it take for 94% of its present radioactivity to decay?

The half-life of X is 3 hours.

Time (Hours)	% of Original Radioactivity
0	100
3	50
6	25
9	12.5
12	6.25

Therefore, after 12 hours, only 6.25% of the original radioactivity remains and approximately 94% has decayed.

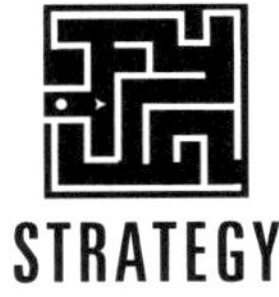

On some MCAT problems dealing with half-life, it may be easier to work backward from the choices. Otherwise, working backward can serve as a method to double-check your answers.

HIGH-YIELD FACTS

19 ESSENTIAL PHYSICS FORMULAS

$$x = x_0 + v_0 t + \tfrac{1}{2} at^2$$
$$v = v_0 + at$$
$$v^2 = v_0^2 + 2as$$

a = acceleration (m/s^2)
s = distance traveled (m)
x = current position (m)
t = time (sec)
v = current velocity (m/s)
x_0 = initial position (m)
v_0 = initial velocity (m/s)

$$slope = \frac{\Delta v}{\Delta t} = a$$

$$v_x = v_0 \cos(\theta)$$
$$v_y = v_0 \sin(\theta)$$

v_x = velocity in the horizontal direction (m/s)
v_y = velocity in the vertical direction (m/s)
v_0 = initial speed of the object (m/s)
θ = angle between the vector v_0 and the horizontal plane

$$F = ma$$

F = force (newtons, N, or kg·m/s^2)
m = mass (kg)
a = acceleration (m/s^2)

and

$$a_c = \frac{v^2}{r}$$
$$F_c = m \times \frac{v^2}{r}$$

a_c = centripetal acceleration (m/s^2)
F_c = centripetal force (N)
m = mass of object (kg)
r = radius of the circular path (m)
v = velocity of object (m/s)

$$F_g = G\frac{m_1 m_2}{r^2}$$

F_g = gravitational force (N)
m_1, m_2 = mass of each object (kg)
r = distance between the 2 objects (m)
G = universal gravitational constant (7×10^{-11} N·m^2/kg^2)

$$F = mg\sin(\theta) = ma$$
$$a = g\sin(\theta)$$

F = force on the object sliding down ramp (N)
g = gravitational constant (9.8 m/s^2)
a = acceleration (m/s^2)
m = mass of the object (kg)
θ = angle between the inclined plane and the horizontal axis

$$f = \mu mg\cos(\theta) = \mu F_N$$

f = frictional force (N)
m = mass of object (kg)
θ = angle between the inclined plane and the horizontal axis
μ = coefficient of friction
g = gravitational constant (9.8 m/s^2)
F_N = normal force acting on the object (N)

$$F = -kx$$

F = force (N)
k = spring constant (N/m)
x = displacement (m)

$$E = \frac{k}{2}x^2$$

E = total energy (N·m)
k = spring constant (N/m)
x = displacement (m)

$$T = 2\pi\sqrt{\frac{l}{g}}$$

T = period of motion (s)
l = length of pendulum (m)
g = gravitational constant (9.8 m/s^2)

$$T = 2\pi\sqrt{\frac{m}{k}}$$

T = period of motion (s)
m = mass at the end of the spring (kg)
k = spring constant (N/m)

$$y_{max} = y_0 + \left|\frac{(v_{0y})^2}{2g}\right|$$

y_{max} = maximum vertical height of projectile (m)
y_0 = initial height from which the projectile was launched (m)
v_{0y} = vertical component of the initial velocity of the projectile (m/s)
g = gravitational constant (9.8 m/s^2)

$$W = F \times d$$

W = work (J)
F = force (N)
d = distance (m)

$$KE = \frac{1}{2} mv^2$$

KE = kinetic energy (J)
m = mass (kg)
v = velocity (m/s)

$$PE = mgh$$

PE = potential energy (J)
m = mass (kg)
g = gravitational constant (9.8 m/s^2)
h = height (m)

$$PE + KE = \text{constant}$$

$$P = \frac{W}{t} = F \times v$$

P = power (watts)
W = work (J)
t = time (s)
F = force (N)
v = velocity (m/s)

$$\begin{aligned} KE_{bottom} &= PE_{top} \\ \frac{1}{2} mv^2 &= mgh \\ v &= \sqrt{2gh} \end{aligned}$$

$$p = mv$$

p = momentum (kg·m/s)
m = mass (kg)
v = velocity (m/s)

$$i = F\Delta t = \Delta p$$

i = impulse (kg·m/s)
F = force (N)
Δp = change in momentum (kg·m/s)
Δt = duration (s)

$$\tau = F \times r$$

τ = torque (N·m)
F = force (N)
r = radius (m)

$$v = f \cdot \lambda$$

v = velocity (m/s)
f = frequency (Hz)
λ = wavelength (m)

$$V = 10 \log\left(\frac{I}{I_0}\right) \qquad \Delta V = 10 \log \frac{I_{new}}{I_{old}}$$

V = volume of sound (dB)
I = intensity of the sound at a given point (W/m^2)
I_0 = threshold of hearing (10^{-12} W/m^2)
I_{new} = new sound intensity (W/m^2)
I_{old} = original sound intensity (W/m^2)

$$\theta_{incident} = \theta_{reflected}$$

$$n_r \sin(\theta_r) = n_i \sin(\theta_i)$$

n_r, n_i = indices of refraction of the refractive and incident media
θ_r, θ_i = angle of the refracted and incident rays with respect to a plane perpendicular to the reflecting surface

$$\sin(\theta_{critical}) = \frac{n_r}{n_i}$$

$\theta_{critical}$ = critical angle
n_r, n_i = indices of refraction of the refractive and incident media

$$\frac{1}{f} = \frac{1}{d_o} + \frac{1}{d_i} = \frac{2}{r}$$

f = focal length of lens (m)
d_i = distance of the image from the lens (m)
d_o = distance of the object from the lens (m)
r = radius of curvature of the lens (m)

$$M = \frac{-d_i}{d_o} = \frac{h_i}{h_o}$$

M = magnification ratio
d_i = distance of image (m)
d_o = distance of object (always positive, m)
h_i = height of image (m)
h_o = height of object (m)

$$D = \frac{1}{f}$$

D = diopter (m^{-1})
f = focal length (m)

$$f_{beat} = |f_1 - f_2|$$

f_{beat} = beat frequency (Hz)
f_1, f_2 = frequencies of overlapping waves (Hz)

$$f' = f\,\frac{v \pm v_d}{v \mp v_s}$$

f' = new frequency (Hz)
f = original frequency (Hz)
v_s = velocity of sound source (m/s)
v_d = velocity of sound detector (m/s)

$$P = \frac{F}{A}$$

P = pressure (pascals [Pa = N/m^2])
F = force (newtons, N)
A = area (m^2)

$$\Delta P = \Phi \cdot R$$

ΔP = change in pressure
Φ = flow
R = resistance

$$R = \frac{8\eta L}{r^4}$$

R = resistance
L = length
η = viscosity
r = radius

$$A_1 v_1 = A_2 v_2$$

A_1, A_2 = cross-sectional area of the entering and leaving streamline bundle
v_1, v_2 = flow velocity in the entering and exiting streamline bundle

$$P + \rho g h + \tfrac{1}{2}\rho v^2 = \text{constant}$$

P = pressure
g = gravitational constant
v = flow velocity
ρ = density
h = height

$$F = qE$$

F = force (N)
q = charge (coulombs)
E = electric field strength (volts/m, V/m)

$$V = \frac{W}{q}$$

$$V = IR$$

V = voltage (volts, V)
I = current (amperes, amp)
R = resistance (ohms, Ω)
W = work (J)
q = charge (coulombs)

$$P = IV = I^2 R = \frac{V^2}{R}$$

P = power (watts, W)
V = voltage (volts, V)
I = current (amperes, amp)
R = resistance (ohms, Ω)

$$R = \frac{\rho_0 L}{A}$$

R = resistance (ohms, Ω)
L = wire length (m)
ρ_0 = resistivity (property of the wire material)
A = cross-sectional area of the wire (m^2)

Resistors in series

$$R_{eq} = R_1 + R_2 + R_3$$

Resistors in parallel

$$\frac{1}{R_{eq}} = \frac{1}{R_1} + \frac{1}{R_2} + \frac{1}{R_3}$$

$$C = \varepsilon_0 \frac{A}{d}$$

C = capacitance (farads, F)
A = plate area
ε_0 = dielectric constant of the medium between the two plates
d = distance separating the plates

$$q = CV$$

$$V = Ed$$

q = charge (coulombs)
C = capacitance
V = voltage
E = electric field strength (V/m)
d = distance (m)

Capacitors in series

$$\frac{1}{C_{eq}} = \frac{1}{C_1} + \frac{1}{C_2} + \frac{1}{C_3}$$

Capacitors in parallel

$$C_{eq} = C_1 + C_2 + C_3$$

$$F = ILB\sin(\theta)$$

F = force (N)
L = length of wire (m)
θ = angle between vector r and wire
I = current (amp)
B = strength of the magnetic field (gauss)

$$E = hf = h\frac{c}{\lambda}$$

E = energy of light (J)
f = frequency (Hz)
λ = wavelength of light (m)
h = Planck's constant
c = speed of light (m/s)

$$E = mc^2$$

E = energy
m = mass
c = speed of light

$$\frac{A}{A_0} = \left(\frac{1}{2}\right)^{t/t_{1/2}}$$

A = number of particles
$t_{1/2}$ = half-life
A_0 = initial number of particles
t = time

E Inorganic Chemistry

1 PERIODIC TRENDS

a. Atomic Radius

- The **metallic atomic radius** is half the distance between the centers of neighboring atoms in a solid sample.
- The **ionic radius** is the distance between the center and the edge of an ion measured in different species.
- **Atomic radius** increases down a column and decreases across a row of the periodic table (Figure 2-8).
- Until you reach the noble gases at the end, the elements on the left are larger than the elements on the right.

b. Electronegativity

- Electronegativity is the ability of an atom to attract electrons in a chemical bond.
- Electronegativity predicts the type of bonding that occurs within a molecule (see Part II E 2).
- Electronegativity increases across a row and decreases down a column of the periodic table (Figure 2-9).
- Electronegativity increases across the periodic table, because more valence electrons are being added and the atom is approaching a stable noble gas electron configuration.
- Electronegativity is inversely related to an atom's atomic radius.

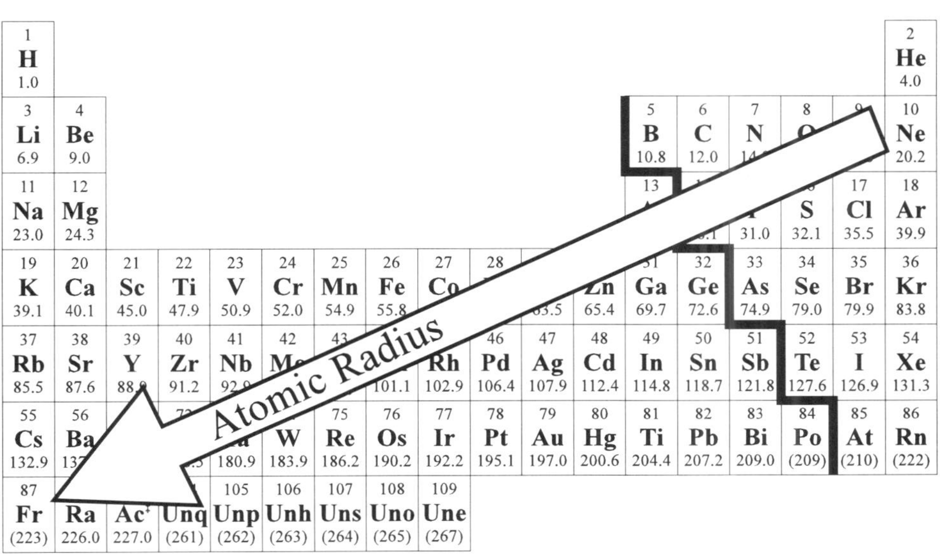

Figure 2-8.
Periodic trend for atomic radius.

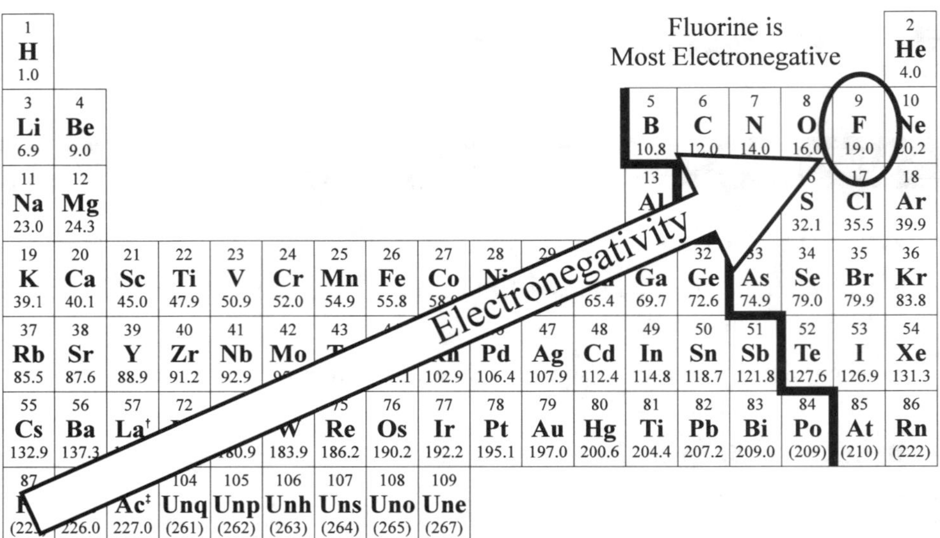

Figure 2-9.
Periodic trend for electronegativity.

- Electronegativity decreases down a column of the periodic table because electrons are dispersing and the nucleus is farther away from free electrons (electric force decreases with the square of the distance).

c. Ionization Energy

- Ionization energy is the minimum energy required to remove an electron from the ground state of a gaseous atom.
- Ionization energy increases across a row and decreases down a column of the periodic table (Figure 2-10).
- The farther the electron is from the nucleus, the easier it is to remove that electron.

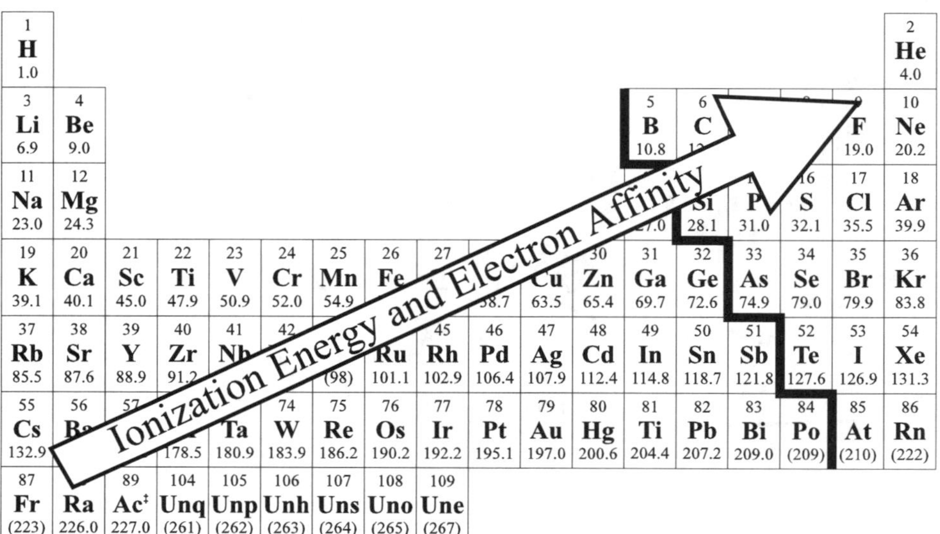

Figure 2-10.
Periodic trend for ionization energy and electron affinity.

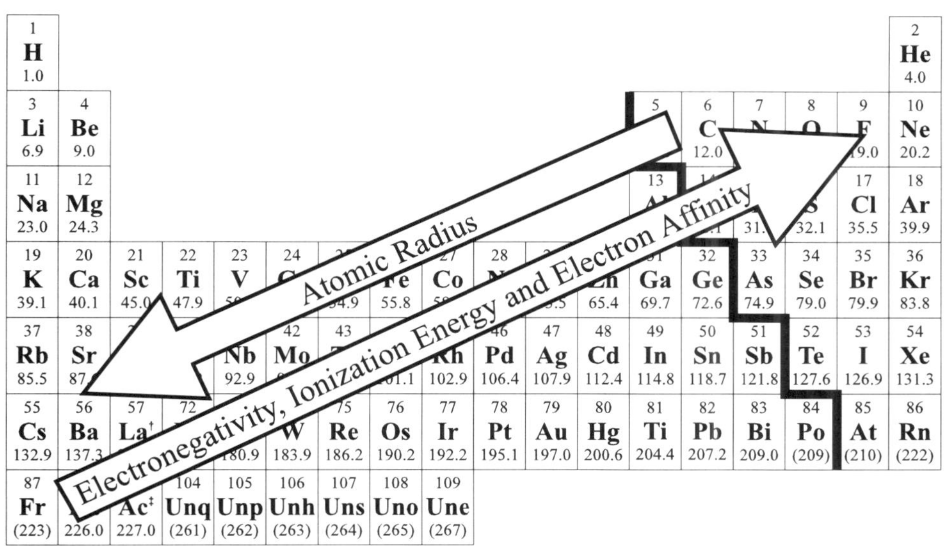

Figure 2-11.
Periodic trends: the big picture.

d. Electron Affinity

- Electron affinity is the amount of energy released when a neutral atom acquires an electron.
- Electron affinity increases across a row and decreases down a column of the periodic table (Figure 2-11).

2 BONDING: INTRAMOLECULAR VERSUS INTERMOLECULAR FORCES

a. Intramolecular Forces

Intramolecular forces (forces within a molecule) are stronger than intermolecular forces (forces between two similar molecules). The type of intramolecular bond between two atoms depends on the electronegativity difference between the two atoms.

1. Covalent bonds

Covalent bonds involve sharing of electrons for atoms of low electronegativity difference (approximately 0.0–1.7). Because of their lower electronegativity difference, covalent bonds are weaker than ionic bonds.

(a) The electronegativity difference of **nonpolar covalent bonds (weak)** is less than 0.4 (e.g., O_2).

(b) The electronegativity difference of **polar covalent bonds (stronger)** is approximately 0.4–1.7 (e.g., H_2O).

2. **Ionic bonds**

Ionic bonds are the strongest chemical bonds (e.g., $Na^{+}Cl^{-}$).

The electronegativity difference of ionic bonds is greater than 1.7.

Ionic bonds involve actual transfer of electrons from one atom to another when forming a chemical bond, because the electronegativity difference is high.

In the solid state, ionic compounds form crystals; in water, they dissolve (at least slightly) to form solutions.

b. Intermolecular Forces

1. **Hydrogen bonding (Figure 2-12)**

In compounds hydrogen bonding occurs only between hydrogen atoms and nitrogen (N), oxygen (O), or fluorine (F) atoms; the hydrogen "latches on" to the N, O, or F because all three have nonbonding electron pairs (e.g., H_2O, HF, NH_3).

Hydrogen bond

:Ö—H·······:Ö: (with H atoms attached to each O)

Figure 2-12. Hydrogen bonding.

In liquids with hydrogen bonding, the additional intermolecular attraction results in a higher boiling point than a non–hydrogen-bonded compound, such as a hydrocarbon of similar molecular weight (e.g., water and ammonia have much higher boiling points than methane).

2. **Van der Waals (dispersion) forces**

Van der Waals forces are the weakest chemical forces; they are found on covalently bonded atoms that have a small (or zero) difference in electronegativity (e.g., H_2, N_2, O_2). These forces result from the constant movement of electrons, which sets up temporary differences in polarity within a nonpolar molecule. Van der Waals forces cause a temporary dipole between two nonpolar molecules. Figure 2-13 is a mnemonic about bond strength.

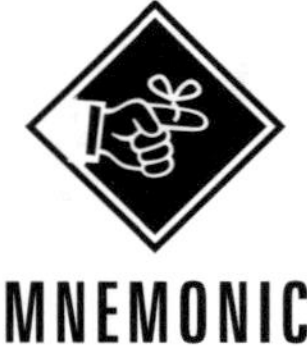

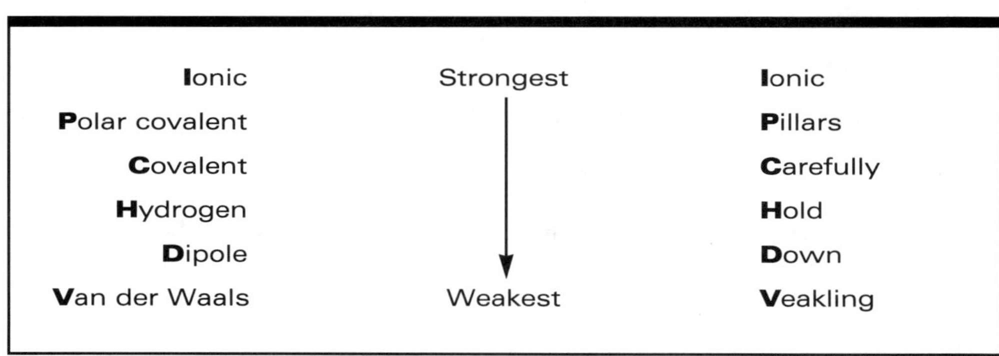

Ionic	Strongest	**I**onic
Polar covalent	↓	**P**illars
Covalent	↓	**C**arefully
Hydrogen	↓	**H**old
Dipole	↓	**D**own
Van der Waals	Weakest	**V**eakling

Figure 2-13. Bond strength mnemonic.

c. Formal charge

is the charge that an individual atom bears in an ion or molecule. Remember the following formula:

Formal charge = valence number of the neutral atom − (dots + bonds).

Determine the formal charge for the following:
(a) The aluminum atom in the compound $AlCl_3$
(b) The carbon atom in formic acid (HCOOH)
(c) The oxygen atom in the hydronium ion (H_3O^+)
(d) The nitrogen atom in glycine at a pH of 1

$\left[\begin{array}{l} H_2CNH_3 \\ \quad | \\ \ \ COOH \end{array}\right]$ Glycine

To determine the formal charge of an atom, first draw the Lewis structure of the ion or molecule and then apply the formula in Part II E 2 c.

(a) 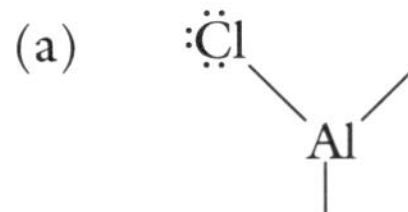

Formal charge of the aluminum atom = 3 − (0 + 3) = 0

(b) 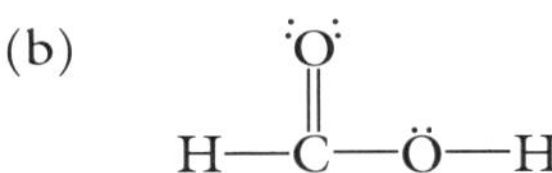

Formal charge of the carbon atom = 4 − (0 + 4) = 0

(c) 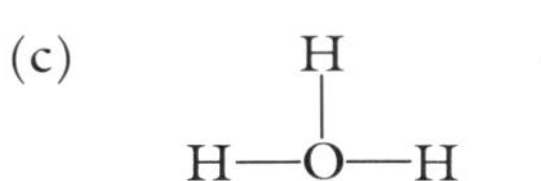

Formal charge of the oxygen atom = 6 − (2 + 3) = + 1

(d) 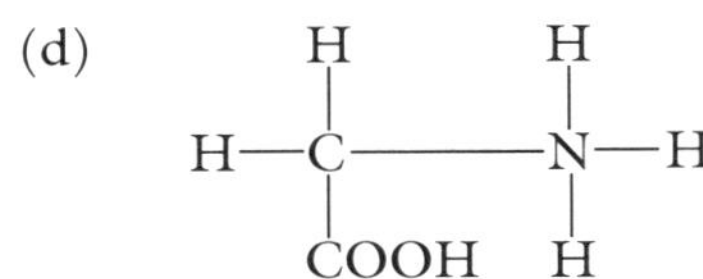

Formal charge of the nitrogen atom = 5 − (0 + 4) = + 1

3 MOLES AND STOICHIOMETRY

A **mole** is a unit of measure equal to 6.02×10^{23} atoms or molecules.

$$\text{Moles} = \frac{\text{grams of molecules}}{\text{molecular weight}}$$

Just as 1 dozen donuts always means 12 donuts, 1 mole of atoms (or molecules) is a constant 6.02×10^{23} atoms (or molecules). The concept of moles is used in calculations of the ideal gas law and solution stoichiometries.

QUESTION

Given the reaction

$$C_3H_8 + 5\ O_2 \Leftrightarrow 3\ CO_2 + 4\ H_2O$$

If 88 g of propane (C_3H_8) [MW = 44 g/mol] combust with excess oxygen, how many grams of water are produced?

ANSWER

$$\frac{88\ \text{g}}{44\ \frac{\text{g}}{\text{mole } C_3H_8}} = 2 \text{ moles of propane}$$

With excess O_2, propane (C_3H_8) is the limiting reagent. In terms of the reaction, each mole of propane combusted produces 4 moles of water. Therefore, 2 moles of propane produce 8 moles of water.

$$8 \text{ moles } H_2O \times 18\ \frac{\text{g}}{\text{mole } H_2O} = 144 \text{ grams of } H_2O$$

4 QUANTUM NUMBERS

a. Definitions

- The **principal quantum number** is n.

  The number of electrons in each principal quantum level = $2n^2$.

- The **angular momentum quantum number** is l.

  l ranges from 0 to (n − 1).

  s: $l = 0$ (The s subshell holds 2 electrons and is spherical.)

  p: $l = 1$ (The p subshell holds 6 electrons and is dumbbell-shaped.)

  d: $l = 2$ (The d subshell holds 10 electrons and includes the transition metal elements.)

  f: $l = 4$ (The f subshell holds 14 electrons and includes the actinides and lanthanides.)

- The **magnetic quantum number** is m_l.

  m_l ranges from $+l$ to $-l$. Each orbital holds two electrons.

- The **spin quantum number** is m_s.

  m_s equals either +1/2 or −1/2. Paired electrons in a given orbital must have opposite spin.

b. Hund's Rule

When electrons fill orbitals of the same energy level, they fill all empty orbitals in the lowest unfilled subshell before entering a half-filled orbital. Because all electrons are negatively charged, they avoid inhabiting the same orbital as long as possible.

c. Pauli's Exclusion Principle

No 2 electrons can share the same set of 4 quantum numbers, and no 2 electrons of identical spin can share the same orbital. The order of filling the orbitals follows the diagonal rule—1s, 2s, 2p, 3s, 3p, 4s, 3d, 4p, 5s, 4d, 5p, 6s, and so forth (Figure 2-14).

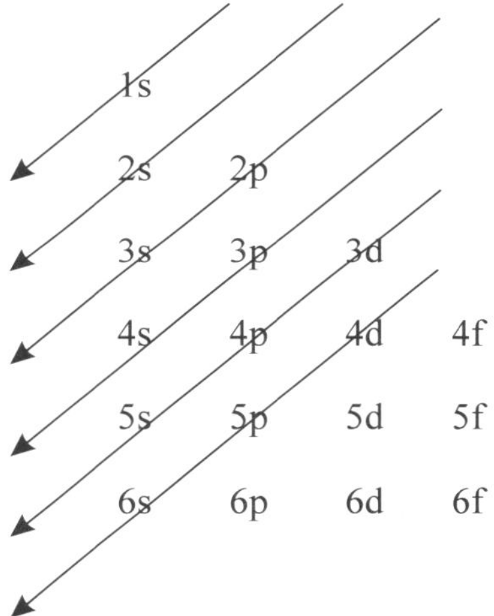

Figure 2-14. Diagonal rule.

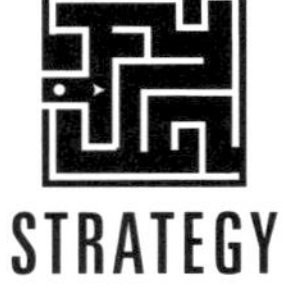

The periodic table (Figure 2-15) organizes the elements according to their respective quantum numbers. For example, the horizontal rows of the periodic table correspond to the principal quantum number. Therefore, carbon and oxygen, which sit in the second row of the periodic table, share the same principal quantum number ($n = 2$). In addition, all the transition metals have occupied d subshells.

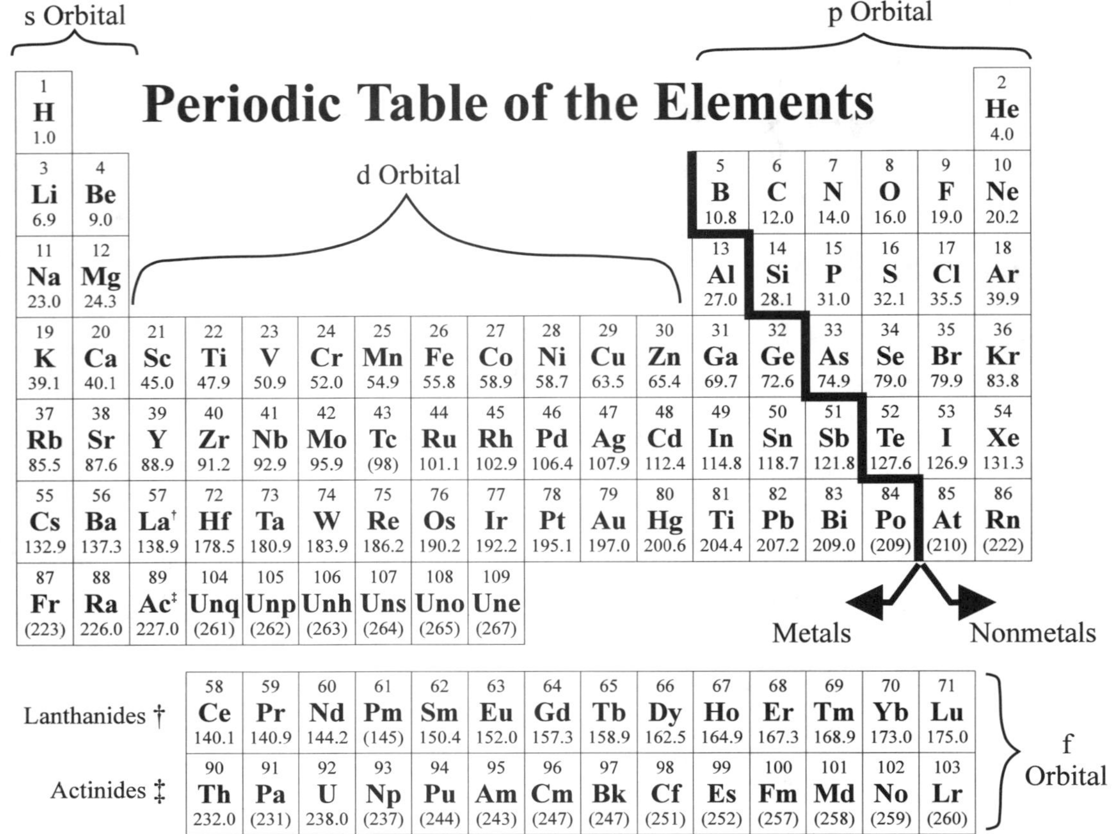

1 H 1.0																	2 He 4.0
3 Li 6.9	4 Be 9.0											5 B 10.8	6 C 12.0	7 N 14.0	8 O 16.0	9 F 19.0	10 Ne 20.2
11 Na 23.0	12 Mg 24.3											13 Al 27.0	14 Si 28.1	15 P 31.0	16 S 32.1	17 Cl 35.5	18 Ar 39.9
19 K 39.1	20 Ca 40.1	21 Sc 45.0	22 Ti 47.9	23 V 50.9	24 Cr 52.0	25 Mn 54.9	26 Fe 55.8	27 Co 58.9	28 Ni 58.7	29 Cu 63.5	30 Zn 65.4	31 Ga 69.7	32 Ge 72.6	33 As 74.9	34 Se 79.0	35 Br 79.9	36 Kr 83.8
37 Rb 85.5	38 Sr 87.6	39 Y 88.9	40 Zr 91.2	41 Nb 92.9	42 Mo 95.9	43 Tc (98)	44 Ru 101.1	45 Rh 102.9	46 Pd 106.4	47 Ag 107.9	48 Cd 112.4	49 In 114.8	50 Sn 118.7	51 Sb 121.8	52 Te 127.6	53 I 126.9	54 Xe 131.3
55 Cs 132.9	56 Ba 137.3	57 La† 138.9	72 Hf 178.5	73 Ta 180.9	74 W 183.9	75 Re 186.2	76 Os 190.2	77 Ir 192.2	78 Pt 195.1	79 Au 197.0	80 Hg 200.6	81 Ti 204.4	82 Pb 207.2	83 Bi 209.0	84 Po (209)	85 At (210)	86 Rn (222)
87 Fr (223)	88 Ra 226.0	89 Ac‡ 227.0	104 Unq (261)	105 Unp (262)	106 Unh (263)	107 Uns (264)	108 Uno (265)	109 Une (267)									

Lanthanides †	58 Ce 140.1	59 Pr 140.9	60 Nd 144.2	61 Pm (145)	62 Sm 150.4	63 Eu 152.0	64 Gd 157.3	65 Tb 158.9	66 Dy 162.5	67 Ho 164.9	68 Er 167.3	69 Tm 168.9	70 Yb 173.0	71 Lu 175.0
Actinides ‡	90 Th 232.0	91 Pa (231)	92 U 238.0	93 Np (237)	94 Pu (244)	95 Am (243)	96 Cm (247)	97 Bk (247)	98 Cf (251)	99 Es (252)	100 Fm (257)	101 Md (258)	102 No (259)	103 Lr (260)

Figure 2-15.
Quantum number arrangement in the periodic table.

1. Which of the following sets of quantum numbers could represent the *first* electron ionized from a calcium atom in its ground state?

	n	l	m_l	m_s
(a)	3	2	2	$-\frac{1}{2}$
(b)	3	3	1	$-\frac{1}{2}$
(c)	4	0	0	$+\frac{1}{2}$
(d)	4	1	1	$+\frac{1}{2}$

2. Write the correct electron configuration for Cu^+ in its ground state.
3. Which ion contains three electrons in its d orbital?

   (a) N^{3-}
   (b) Mn^{2+}
   (c) Ni^+
   (d) Cu^+

ANSWER

1. The answer is (c). In any given atom, the first electron to be ionized is the one in the outermost shell. Because calcium has an atomic number of 20, its electron configuration in its ground state is $1s^2\ 2s^2\ 2p^6\ 3s^2\ 3p^6\ 4s^2$. Thus, the electrons in its outermost shell are in the $4s^2$ orbital, where $n = 4$, $l = 0$, $m_l = 0$, and $m_s = \pm\frac{1}{2}$.
2. Because Cu^+ has +1 charge, the atom has lost one electron, leaving it with a positive charge. Thus, if the atomic number of copper is 29, Cu^+ has 28 electrons. The two electrons in the 4s orbital move to fill the last vacant 3d orbital, resulting in increased stability. Therefore, the electron configuration of Cu^+ in the ground state is $1s^2\ 2s^2 2p^6 3s^2 3p^6 4s^0 3d^{10}$. This exception in the order of electron filling occurs with Cr, Cu, and Ag atoms because a half-filled (d=5) or completely filled (d=10) d subshell provides added stability.
3. The answer is (b). Looking at the periodic table, you can see the transitional metals represent atoms with electrons in their d orbital. Therefore, atoms or ions with three electrons in their d orbitals have atomic numbers of 23, 41, 73, and 105. Thus, the best way to solve this problem is to figure out the number of electrons of the ions listed. Remember: Number of electrons = atomic number − (charge of ion).

N^{3-} Number of electrons = 7 − (−3) = 10 electrons

Mn^{2+} Number of electrons = 25 − (+2) = 23 electrons

Ni^+ Number of electrons = 28 − (+1) = 27 electrons

Cu^{2+} Number of electrons = 29 − (+2) = 27 electrons

Thus, Mn^{2+} has 3 electrons in its d orbitals.

QUESTION

Why are aqueous ionic solutions of transition metals (e.g., Fe^{3+}, Cu^{2+}) colored?

ANSWER

Aqueous ionic solutions of transition metals often have 1 or more electrons in the ground state of an unfilled high-energy d orbital; therefore, these transition metal electrons can absorb light energy and enter into an excited state. For example, an electron in the 4s subshell of Fe^{3+} (ground state: $1s^2 2s^2 2p^6 3s^2 3p^6 4s^2 3d^3$) can absorb a photon of appropriate energy to enter into a higher energy orbital in the 3d subshell (excited state: $1s^2 2s^2 2p^6 3s^2 3p^6 4s^1 3d^4$). When this electron returns to its ground state (goes back to its lower energy 4s subshell), it emits this lost energy in the form of light of a higher wavelength and lower energy than that originally absorbed by the electron. This emission of energy appears as a colored solution.

5 IDEAL GAS LAW

The ideal gas law is a combination of three basic laws for ideal gases.

a. Boyle's Law

At constant temperature, the pressure of a gas is inversely proportional to the volume:

$$P_1 V_1 = P_2 V_2 \text{ at constant temperature}$$

b. Charles' Law

At constant pressure, the volume of a gas is directly proportional to the temperature:

$$\frac{V_1}{T_1} = \frac{V_2}{T_2} \text{ at constant pressure}$$

c. Avogadro's Law

At constant pressure and temperature, the volume of a gas is directly proportional to the number of moles of gas:

$$PV = nRT$$

$$PV = \frac{gRT}{MW}$$

$$P = \frac{\rho RT}{MW}$$

$$\frac{P_1 V_1}{T_1} = \frac{P_2 V_2}{T_2}$$

P = pressure (atm)
n = moles of gas
T = absolute temperature (K)
MW = molecular weight (g/mol)
V = volume (L)
R = gas constant (0.0821 L·atm/mol·K)
ρ = density (g/L)
g = grams of gas (g)

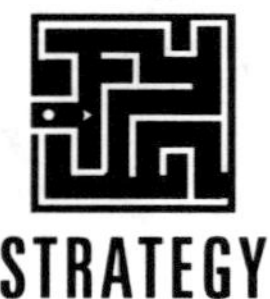
STRATEGY

Estimate before you calculate.

(1) **PV = nRT** is the key form of the ideal gas law to remember because from this equation, you can derive all its variations through the relationships among temperature, pressure, volume, and number of moles (e.g., moles = mass/molecular weight; density = grams/volume).

When doing calculations based on the ideal gas law, **round R to 0.1 L atm/mol K** to save time. Then, **estimate before you calculate.**

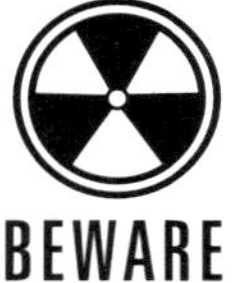
BEWARE

(2) **Standard temperature and pressure** (STP) is defined as 1 atm of pressure at 273 K. At STP, 1 mole of gas occupies 22.4 L. This volume (1 mole gas = 22.4 L) is true **if and only if** the gas is at STP.

The greatest deviation from the ideal gas law occurs when molecules have very low energy (low temperatures) or are very close together (high pressures), because intermolecular (e.g., Van der Waals) forces start affecting these variables.

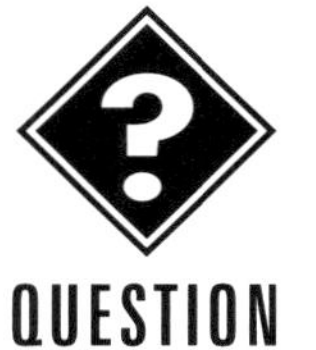
QUESTION

Thirty grams of nitrogen gas (N_2) is placed in a 2-L container at room temperature (25°C).

(a) What is the pressure in atmospheres of the nitrogen gas?
(b) If the temperature has changed to 0°C and the pressure was held constant at 1 atmosphere, what volume would the nitrogen gas occupy?
(c) At *extremely* high pressures and *extremely* low temperatures (e.g., absolute zero), how would nitrogen gas differ in pressure and volume from an ideal gas?

ANSWER

ESTIMATE

use 0.1 for R

(a) $PV = \frac{gRT}{MW}$

$$P = \frac{gRT}{(V)(MW)} = \frac{(30)(0.0821)(298)}{(2)(28)} \approx \frac{(\not{30})(0.1)(300)}{(2)(\not{30})}$$

$= 15$ atm

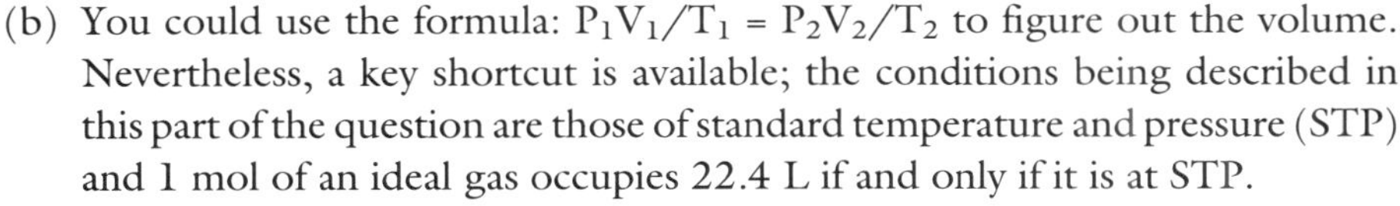
(b) You could use the formula: $P_1V_1/T_1 = P_2V_2/T_2$ to figure out the volume. Nevertheless, a key shortcut is available; the conditions being described in this part of the question are those of standard temperature and pressure (STP) and 1 mol of an ideal gas occupies 22.4 L if and only if it is at STP.

$$\text{moles} = \frac{\text{grams}}{\text{MW}}$$

$$= \frac{30}{28} \approx 1 \text{ mol } N_2 \qquad \frac{22.4 \text{ L}}{1 \text{ mol gas}} \times 1 \text{ mol } N_2 = 22.4 \text{ L}$$

(c) Because Van der Waals forces would cause a repulsive force between molecules of N_2 at small intermolecular distances, the volume would be higher and the pressure would be lower than those of an ideal gas.

6 DALTON'S LAW OF PARTIAL PRESSURES

Dalton's law. For a mixture of gases, the total pressure is the sum of the partial pressures of each of the individual gases in the mixture.

$$P_{total} = P_A + P_B + P_C$$

$$X_A = \frac{\text{moles of A}}{\text{total number of moles}}$$

P_{total} = total pressure
$P_{A,B,C}$ = partial pressures of various components
X_A = mole fraction

Dalton's law of partial pressure expressed in terms of mole fraction is:

$$P_A = P_{total}X_A$$

(Raoult's law; see Part II E 8)

7 MOLARITY, MOLALITY, AND NORMALITY

a. Molarity

The concentration of a specific molecule in a solution can be expressed as a ratio of moles of solute to liters of solution.

$$\text{Molarity (M)} = \frac{\text{moles of solute}}{\text{liters of solution}}$$

b. Molality

The concentration of a specific molecule in a solution can be expressed as a ratio of moles of solute to kilograms of solvent.

$$\text{Molality (m)} = \frac{\text{moles of solute}}{\text{kilograms of solvent}}$$

Molarity and molality of dilute aqueous solutions are roughly equivalent if water is the solvent. Remember that the density of water is 1 g/ml; therefore, 1 L of water weighs 1 kg.

c. Normality

The concentration of a specific molecule in a solution can be expressed as a ratio of solute equivalents (e.g., oxidizing/reducing equivalents, acid/base equivalents) to liters of solution.

$$\text{Normality (N)} = \text{molarity} \times \text{number of equivalents}$$

For example, a 1-molar solution of H_2SO_4, which can donate 2 protons, is a 2-N solution.

d. Dilution Equation

$$M_1 V_1 = M_2 V_2$$

When you dilute an aqueous solution, the number of moles of solute stays constant.

8 COLLIGATIVE PROPERTIES

a. Definition

Physical properties of a solution that depend on the number of particles in the solution are called colligative properties. The four types are:

- Boiling-point elevation: $\Delta T_b = K_b mi$
- Freezing-point depression: $\Delta T_f = K_f mi$
- Osmotic pressure: $P = MRTi$
- Raoult's law: $P_A = P_{total} X_A$

ΔT_b = change in boiling point
K_b = molal boiling-point elevation constant
m = molality
M = molarity
T = temperature (kelvins, K)
P_A = partial pressure of gas A
P_{total} = total pressure of gaseous mixture
ΔT_f = change in freezing point
K_f = molal freezing-point depression constant
i = number of particles per molecule
R = ideal gas law constant (0.08 L/mol K—round to 0.1)
X_A = mole fraction of gas A

b. For Raoult's law,

whenever you put a solid in a liquid, the vapor pressure of the solvent decreases.

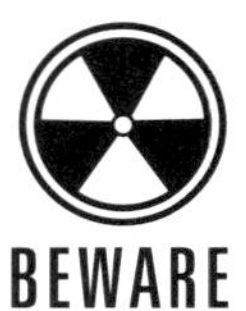

- Remember that the m stands for molality, not molarity.
- Remember to take into account the number of particles in the solution (i).
- The formulas for boiling-point elevation and freezing-point depression give you the **change** in the boiling point and freezing point, respectively. To derive the new freezing point (or the boiling point) of the solution, subtract this number from the freezing point or add this number to the boiling point of the solvent.

$$T_b^{new} = T_b^{pure} + K_b mi$$

$$T_f^{new} = T_f^{pure} - K_f mi$$

QUESTION

Which aqueous solution has the highest boiling point?
(a) 1 molal NaCl
(b) 2 molal $MgCl_2$
(c) 4 molal glucose
(d) 2 molal KCl

ANSWER

The equation to use is:

$$\Delta T_b = K_b m i$$

Because i = 3 for $MgCl_2$ (i.e., $MgCl_2$ splits into 1 Mg^{2+} ion and 2 Cl^- ions) and it is a 2-molal solution, it has the highest boiling-point elevation. Therefore, the correct answer is (b).

9 EQUILIBRIUM: GENERAL CONCEPTS

Equilibrium is the situation or stage when the rate of the forward reaction is equal to the rate of the reverse reaction; at that point, the concentrations of the reactants and products no longer change with time. At equilibrium, $\Delta G = 0$.

In the reaction:

$$aA(aq) + bB(g) + cC(s) \Leftrightarrow dD(aq) + eE(l) + fF(g)$$

$$K_{eq} = \frac{D^d F^f}{A^a B^b}$$

Remember that K_{eq} is the ratio of products over reactants, with the mole coefficient as the exponent. In addition, only gases and aqueous solutions figure into the K_{eq} (not solids or liquids). From the K_{eq}, you can calculate the **Gibbs free energy** (ΔG), using the following relationship:

$$\Delta G = -RT \ln(K_{eq})$$

R = gas constant
T = temperature (K)

10 LE CHATELIER'S PRINCIPLE

Le Chatelier's principle. If the environment changes, the reaction always shifts to a new equilibrium to reduce the stress on the system.

For example, if the temperature of a system increases, the reaction shifts to absorb heat (or vice versa if the temperature decreases). If pressure increases, the reaction shifts to the side that has fewer moles of gas (and the compounds take up less space). If you add more of a reactant or product, the reaction shifts to consume some (but not all) of the added reactant or product.

QUESTION

In the exothermic reaction

$$C_3H_8(g) + 5\ O_2(g) \Leftrightarrow 3\ CO_2(g) + 4H_2O(g)$$

which way does the reaction shift if:
(a) The temperature is increased?
(b) The pressure is increased?
(c) A dehydrating agent is added to the reaction vessel?

ANSWER

(a) The reaction is exothermic; therefore, heat is a product of the reaction.

$$C_3H_8 + 5\ O_2 \Leftrightarrow 3\ CO_2 + 4\ H_2O + \text{heat}$$

If the temperature is increased (i.e., more heat is added), the reaction shifts to the **left.**

(b) If the pressure is increased, the effective volume decreases, and the reaction shifts to the side that has the lower number of moles of gas. In this case, the reaction shifts to the **left.**

(c) If a dehydrating agent is added to the reaction vessel, this agent absorbs all the water. Because you are removing one of the products of the reaction (i.e., water), the reaction shifts to the **right.**

11 PHASE EQUILIBRIA

Phase diagram. Plotting the pressure of a compound versus the temperature for its three basic states (solid, liquid, or gas) lets you predict the conditions for equilibrium among the states of the compound (Figure 2-16).

Water is most dense at 4°C; therefore, an increase in pressure at the triple point favors the liquid phase. This situation explains why segment BC has a negative slope. Carbon dioxide is most dense when it is solid; therefore, segment BC in this diagram has a positive slope. **An increase in pressure at the triple point favors the most dense phase.**

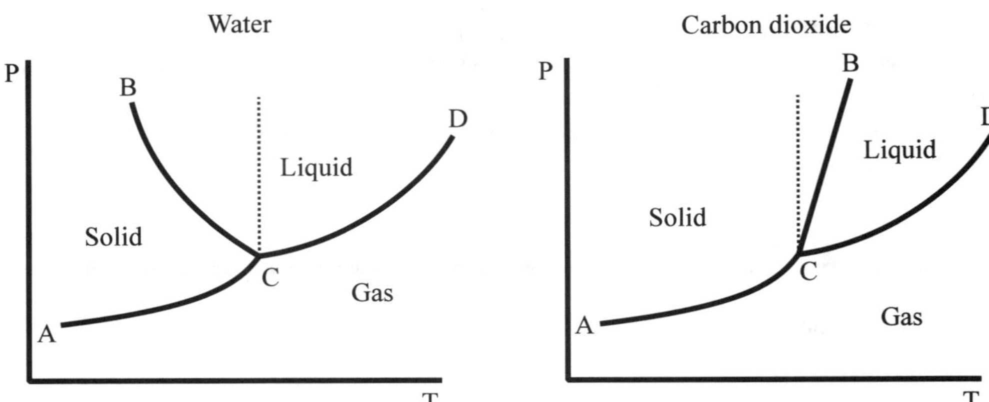

Figure 2-16. Pressure–temperature phase diagrams for water and carbon dioxide. *AC* = sublimation: a phase change from solid to gas that bypasses the liquid phase; *CD* = boiling/condensation; *D* = critical point: the temperature at which a pressure increase can no longer cause condensation; *BC* = freezing/melting; *C* = triple point (solid, liquid, and gas phases coexist in equilibrium): when an increase in pressure favors the densest phase.

12 SOLUBILITY EQUILIBRIA, PRECIPITATION, AND THE COMMON ION EFFECT

a. Solubility equilibria

is the state of equilibrium between the solid form of a compound (precipitate) and its aqueous form in a specific solvent.

$$BaSO_4(s) \Leftrightarrow Ba^{2+}(aq) + SO_4(aq)$$

$$K_{sp} = [Ba^{2+}][SO_4^{2-}]$$

K_{sp} = solubility product constant

Therefore, the lower the K_{sp}, the more insoluble the compound. In nonequilibrium conditions:

$$Q = [Ba^{2+}][SO_4^{2-}]$$

Q = nonequilibrium ion product

Equilibrium is reached when $Q = K_{sp}$.

b. Precipitation

is the formation of an insoluble, solid compound from its ions in solution.

- If $Q > K_{sp}$, the solution precipitates (the gunk settles at the bottom of the beaker).
- If $Q < K_{sp}$, the solution does not precipitate (all of the compound dissolves in solution).

c. Common Ion Effect

A compound is less soluble in a solution that contains an ion identical to one of its dissociation products. Le Chatelier's principle fully explains the common ion effect.

For example, $BaSO_4$ is more soluble in a 1-M NaCl solution than in a 1-M solution of $BaCl_2$ because the Ba^{2+} is an ion present in both the compound and the solvent. The Ba^{2+} in the solvent shifts the reaction to the left, favoring formation of the $BaSO_4$ precipitate.

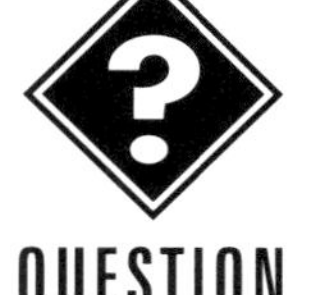

One liter of a 0.05 M Fe^{3+} solution is prepared at a pH of 7. [K_{sp} of $Fe(OH)_3$ = 6.3×10^{-38}]

(a) Will a precipitate form?
(b) At what pH will a precipitate start to form?
(c) Will the addition of HCl increase or decrease the solubility of $Fe(OH)_3$?

(a) For a precipitate to form, Q must be greater than K_{sp}. Thus, to solve this problem, we need to calculate the value of Q:

$$Q = [Fe^{3+}][OH^-]^3$$

$$pOH = 14 - pH = -\log[OH^-]$$

$$pOH = 14 - 7 = -\log[OH^-]$$

$$\text{Concentration of } (OH^-) = 1 \times 10^{-7}$$

$$Q = (5 \times 10^{-2})(1 \times 10^{-7})^3 = 5 \times 10^{-23},$$

which is greater than K_{sp} of 6.3×10^{-38}

Because Q is greater than K_{sp}, a precipitate will form.

(b) A precipitate will start to form as Q becomes greater than K_{sp}. Thus,

$$K_{sp} = 6.3 \times 10^{-38} = [Fe^{3+}][OH^-]^3$$

$$6.3 \times 10^{-38} = [5 \times 10^{-2}][OH^-]^3$$

$$\text{Concentration of } OH^- \text{ when precipitate begins to form} = \sqrt[3]{\frac{6.3 \times 10^{-38}}{5 \times 10^{-2}}} \approx 1 \times 10^{-12}$$

$$pOH = -\log(1 \times 10^{-12}) = 12$$

$$pH = 14 - pOH = 14 - 12 = 2$$

Therefore, a precipitate begins to form when the pH rises above 2.

(c) Look at the solubility reaction:

$$Fe(OH)_3(s) \rightarrow Fe^{3+}(aq) + 3OH^-(aq)$$

Adding HCl will neutralize and decrease the concentration of OH^-. Based on Le Chatelier's principle, decreasing the concentration of OH^- will shift the reaction to the right, thus decreasing the amount of precipitate that is formed.

13 CALORIMETRY AND HEAT TRANSFER

a. Calorimetry

is a technique that permits the measurement of heat absorbed or released from a physical process such as a chemical reaction. A change in phase or temperature can be tracked as a transfer of heat in potential energy.

For simple heating of a compound without a change in phase, use the following equation:

$$q = mc\Delta T$$

c = specific heat: The number of joules or calories it takes to heat 1 gram of a particular compound 1 Kelvin

q = heat added (calories or joules)
m = mass
ΔT = change in temperature

b. Heat Transfer

For the amount of heat added or released from a change in phase of a compound at a specific temperature:

$$q = mL$$

q = heat added (calories or joules)
m = mass
L = latent heat (heat of fusion or vaporization): The number of joules or calories it takes to melt/freeze (equal but opposite in sign) or vaporize/condense (equal but opposite in sign)

A phase change can also happen at constant temperature (see preceding phase diagrams). Heat is still transferred.

$$c_{water} = 1\,\frac{\text{cal}}{\text{g}\cdot{}^\circ\text{C}} = 4.18\,\frac{\text{J}}{\text{g}\cdot{}^\circ\text{C}}$$

c = specific heat of water

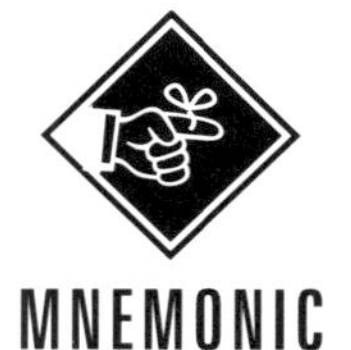

Heat (q) = MCAT (mcΔT). "The heat is on" when you are taking the MCAT.

How much heat does it take to bring 5 g of ice at −10°C to 5 g of steam at 120°C? It is given that the specific heat of water, steam, and ice is 1 kcal/g °C; the heat of fusion of water is 20 kcal/g; and the heat of vaporization of water is 40 kcal/g.

This problem consists of the following steps:

1. Heat ice at −10°C to ice at 0°C

$$q_1 = mc\Delta T = 5 \cdot 1 \cdot 10 = 50 \text{ kcal}$$

2. Heat ice at 0°C to water at 0°C (melting)

$$q_2 = mL = 5 \cdot 20 = 100 \text{ kcal}$$

3. Heat water at 0°C to water at 100°C

$$q_3 = mc\Delta T = 5 \cdot 1 \cdot 100 = 500 \text{ kcal}$$

4. Heat water at 100°C to steam at 100°C (boiling)

$$q_4 = mL = 5 \cdot 40 = 200 \text{ kcal}$$

5. Heat steam at 100°C to steam at 120°C

$$q_5 = mc\Delta T = 5 \cdot 1 \cdot 20 = 100 \text{ kcal}$$

$$q_{total} = q_1 + q_2 + q_3 + q_4 + q_5 = 950 \text{ kcal}$$

14 THERMODYNAMICS

a. Enthalpy (ΔH)

is the change in heat during a reaction that occurs at constant pressure. If a negative ΔH means that the reaction gives off heat (exothermic), a positive ΔH means that the reaction absorbs heat (endothermic).

TABLE 2-3. Free energy of a reaction

If ΔG is	The reaction is
Negative	Spontaneous
Zero	At equilibrium
Positive	Nonspontaneous

b. Entropy (ΔS)

is the amount of unusable energy (disorder) in a reaction. *ΔS* corresponds to the change in the randomness or disorder during a reaction. If *ΔS* is positive, the reaction gets more random and disordered (e.g., the transition from solid to liquid). If it is negative, the reaction gets more ordered.

As a general rule, the **entropy of gases > liquids > solids.**

c. Free energy of a reaction (ΔG)

This quantity tells us whether the reaction is spontaneous (Table 2-3).

d. Gibbs-Helmholtz equation (Table 2-4)

$$\Delta G = \Delta H - T\Delta S$$

ΔG = Gibbs' free energy (J)
ΔH = enthalpy (J)
T = temperature (K)
ΔS = entropy (J/K)

e. Laws of Thermodynamics

1. **First law of thermodynamics.** The first law of thermodynamics states that the internal energy of an isolated system (E) is constant. To change the in-

TABLE 2-4. Dependence of ΔG on the sign and magnitude of ΔH and ΔS

If ΔH is	And ΔS is	ΔG is
Positive	**Negative**	Always positive A nonspontaneous reaction at all temperatures
Negative	**Positive**	Always negative A spontaneous reaction at all temperatures
Positive	**Positive**	Positive at low temperatures Negative at high temperatures
Negative	**Negative**	Negative at low temperatures Positive at high temperatures

ternal energy (E) of a system, you must either do work (w) or add or remove heat (q); and, as a result, the system is no longer isolated.

$$E = q + w$$

2. **Second law of thermodynamics.** In a spontaneous reaction, entropy always increases—as long as you take into account not just the system but the entire environment.
3. **Third law of thermodynamics.** The entropy of a perfect crystal at absolute zero is 0; in other words, a perfect crystal is in perfect order at absolute zero. However, this state can never be attained (i.e., some entropy always exists).

f. Thermodynamics and the Facts of Life

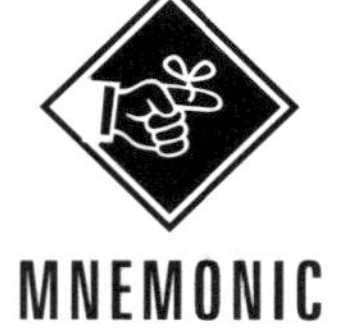

MNEMONIC

The laws of thermodynamics are like the facts of life.

1. **First law of thermodynamics.** A no-win situation. You can never win (get more energy than you put in); you can only break even ($\Delta E = q + w$).
2. **Second law of thermodynamics.** Murphy's law. You will not be lucky enough to break even—you will always lose. (A spontaneous reaction always involves a loss of energy because of an increase in entropy.)
3. **Third law of thermodynamics.** Nobody's perfect. Some entropy is always present (unless you have a perfect crystal at absolute zero).

15 ENTHALPY: HEAT OF FORMATION, BOND ENERGY, AND HESS'S LAW

a. Heat of Formation

The heat of formation (ΔH_f) is the heat of the reaction that produces a compound in its standard state from its elements. The heat of a reaction (ΔH_{rxn}) equals the difference between the product's and the reactant's heat of formation (ΔH_f).

$$\Delta H_{rxn} = \Sigma H_f(\text{products}) - \Sigma H_f(\text{reactants})$$

ΔH (also known as the enthalpy change) signifies the change in enthalpy caused by the reaction. For example, a reaction that gives off 40 kcal per mole of reactant (i.e., raises the temperature of 1 kg of water by 40 degrees) has a ΔH of −40 kcal/mol. For the reaction

$$2A + B \rightarrow A_2B$$

$\Delta H_f A$ = 20 kcal/mol
$\Delta H_f B$ = −10 kcal/mol
$\Delta H_f A_2B$ = 40 kcal/mol

To get ΔH for this reaction, subtract the reactants' heats of formation from the products' heats of formation. Be careful to take into account the number of moles of each product and reactant. ΔH for this reaction would be calculated as follows:

$$\Delta H = \left(40\ \frac{\text{kcal}}{\text{mole}}\right)(1\ \text{mole}) - \left[\left(-10\ \frac{\text{kcal}}{\text{mole}}\right)(1\ \text{mole}) + \left(20\ \frac{\text{kcal}}{\text{mole}}\right)(2\ \text{mole})\right] = 10\ \frac{\text{kcal}}{\text{mole}}$$

b. Hess's law

states that ΔHs are additive; therefore:

$$X \xrightarrow{\Delta H = a} Y$$

$$Y \xrightarrow{\Delta H = b} Z$$

$$X \xrightarrow{\Delta H = a+b} Z$$

c. Calculating ΔH from Bond Energies

Breaking bonds is an endothermic process ($\Delta H > 0$) requiring an input of energy. Forming bonds is an exothermic process ($\Delta H < 0$) involving the release of heat. You can use bond enthalpies or energies (the two terms are used interchangeably) to calculate the enthalpy of a reaction. Look at the following reaction:

$$CH_3OH(g) + \tfrac{3}{2}O_2(g) \rightarrow CO_2(g) + 2H_2O$$

The heat required to break the bonds of the reactants:

$$\Delta H = 3\cdot(\text{C—H}) + (\text{C—O}) + \tfrac{3}{2}\cdot(\text{O=O}) + (\text{O—H})$$

$$\Delta H = 3\cdot(412\ \text{kJ}) + 360\ \text{kJ} + \tfrac{3}{2}\cdot(498\ \text{kJ}) + 463\ \text{kJ} = 2806\ \text{kJ}$$

The heat released when the new bonds form to make the products:

$$\Delta H = 2\cdot(\text{C=O}) + 4\cdot(\text{O—H})$$

$$\Delta H = 2\cdot(803\ \text{kJ}) + 4\cdot(463\ \text{kJ}) = 3458\ \text{kJ}$$

$$\Delta H = (\text{Heat needed to break bonds}) - (\text{Heat released when making bonds})$$

$$\Delta H = 2806\ \text{kJ} - 3458\ \text{kJ} = -652\ \frac{\text{kJ}}{\text{mole}}\ CH_3OH$$

16 CHEMICAL KINETICS

Activation energy. The minimum kinetic energy needed for a reaction to proceed (Figure 2-17). The activation energy allows reactants to progress to the transition state (D) of a reaction before yielding products.

As Figure 2-17 shows, enzymes (biological catalysts) and other catalysts increase the rate of the reaction by lowering the activation energy of **both** the forward and re-

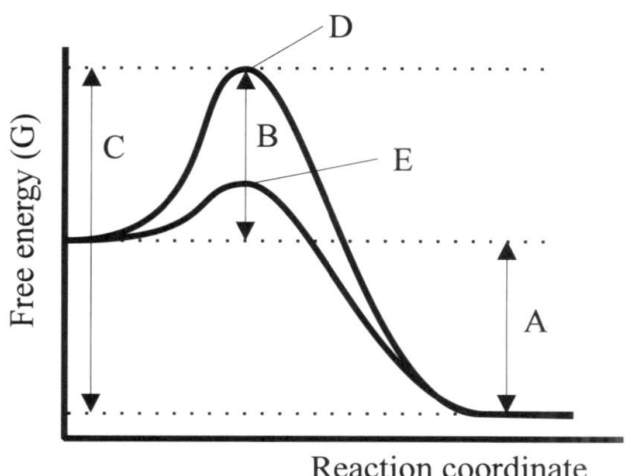

Figure 2-17.
Activation energy diagram. *A* = ΔG of the reaction; here, ΔG is negative, so the reaction is spontaneous; a reaction with a positive ΔG is nonspontaneous. *B* = activation energy of the forward reaction. *C* = activation energy of the reverse reaction. *D* = transition state (activated complex); it is the most unstable arrangement of atoms/molecules in the reaction. *E* = path of the catalyzed or enzymatic reaction.

verse reactions, but they do **not** change *ΔG*.

A rise in temperature, which means an increased number of molecular collisions (increased kinetic energy), results in an increased rate of reaction.

A reaction proceeds along a reaction coordinate from reactants to products.

QUESTION

For the reaction

$$A + B \rightarrow C$$

the following data were obtained:

Experiment No.	[A]	[B]	Rate
1	0.35	0.20	3.0
2	0.70	0.20	12.0
3	0.35	0.40	6.0
4	0.70	0.40	24.0

What is the rate law for this reaction?

ANSWER

Comparing reactions 1 and 2 shows that as the concentration of A doubles, (whereas the concentration of B remained constant), the rate of reaction increases fourfold. The rate order with respect to reactant A is calculated by solving for n in the equation $2^n = 4$. Here, the rate order (n) is 2. In comparing reactions 1 and 3, as the concentration of B doubles (whereas the concentration of A remains constant), the rate of reaction increases twofold. Therefore, the rate order with respect to reactant B is 1 ($2^n = 2$). **Therefore, the rate = $k[A]^2[B]$, and the overall order for the reaction is 3.**

17 REDOX REACTIONS AND VOLTAIC/ELECTROLYTIC CELLS

a. Redox reactions

involve the oxidation and reduction (transfer of electrons) of reactants in the formation of products.

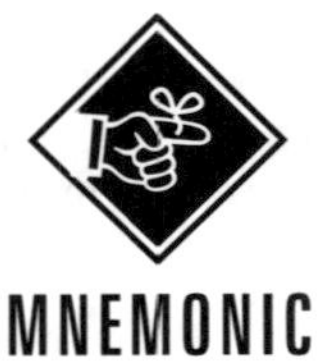

"**Leo** says **Ger**."

Loss of **e**lectrons is **o**xidation; **g**ain in **e**lectrons is **r**eduction.

b. Voltaic Cell

In a voltaic cell, anion flow goes from anode to cathode.

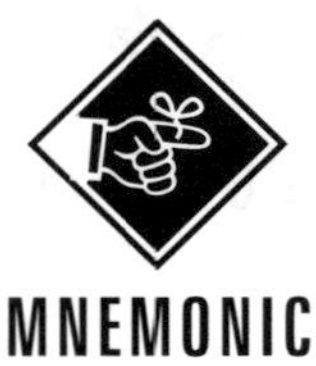

"**An Ox** and **red cat**."

Oxidation occurs at the **an**ode (−); **red**uction occurs at the **cat**hode (+).

c. Electrolytic Cell

In an electrolytic cell, anions migrate to the anode and cations migrate to the cathode (i.e., electron flow is opposite that of a voltaic cell) [Figure 2-18]

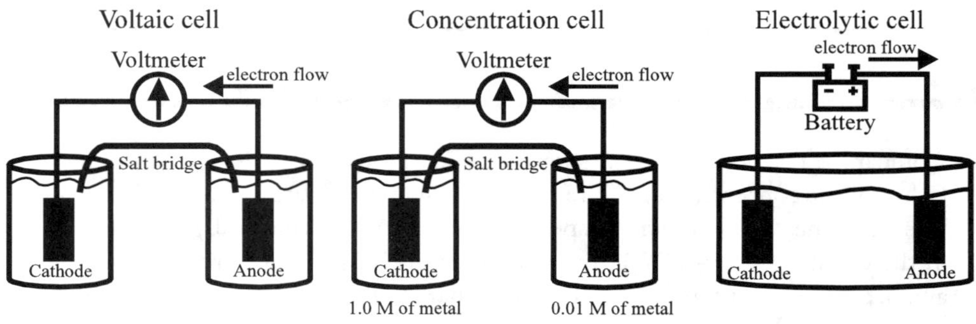

Figure 2-18.
Voltaic versus electrolytic cell.

18 REDOX, NERNST EQUATION, AND FREE ENERGY

The **Nernst equation** relates the voltage E derived from a voltaic cell to the free energy ΔG and equilibrium constant K_{eq} of the chemical reaction driving the battery:

$$E_{cell} = E^0 - \frac{0.06}{n}\log(Q)$$

E_{cell} = voltage derived from a chemical battery
n = number of electrons transferred in the redox reaction
Q = nonequilibrium ion product (mass action expression for the chemical battery reaction)
E^0 = standard reduction potential for the voltaic cell (all reactants and products at 1 M)

$$\Delta G = -nFE$$
$$= -RT\ln(K_{eq})$$

n = charge of the ionic species in solution
F = Faraday's constant, 96,500 coul/mol of electrons
T = temperature (Kelvin)
R = 8.31 J/K
K_{eq} = equilibrium constant of the reaction

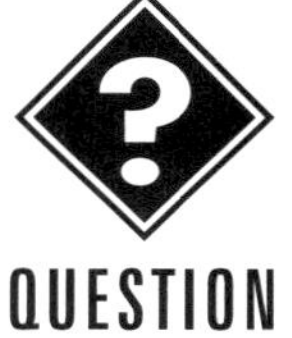

A 10-amp battery is used to drive the following half-reaction:

$$Au^{2+}(aq) + 2e \rightarrow Au(s)$$

The battery is connected to this circuit, which runs for 30 minutes. How much solid gold is formed?

To answer this question, you must know the definition of a coulomb (coul).

1 coulomb = a unit of charge = (1 amp)(sec)

Therefore, in this reaction:

charge = (10 amp)(30 min)(60 sec/min) = 18,000 coul

Now, use Faraday's law to determine the moles of electrons produced:

[(18,000 coul)/(96,500 coul/mol electron)] = ~0.2 mol electrons

Then use stoichiometry to derive the moles of gold formed:

0.2 mol electrons × (1 mol Au/2 mol e^-) = 0.1 mol Au (s)

To find the mass (grams) of gold formed, multiply the moles of gold by its molecular weight:

0.1 mol Au × 197 g/mol = ~20 g of solid gold formed

19 ACID-BASE DEFINITIONS

TABLE 2-5. Definition of acid and base

Chemical Type	Arrhenius Definition	Bronsted-Lowry Definition	Lewis Definition
Acid	Produces H^+ or H_3O^+ upon dissociation in water	H^+ (proton) donor	Electron (e^-) acceptor
Base	Produces OH^- upon dissociation in water	H^+ (proton) acceptor	Electron (e^-) donor

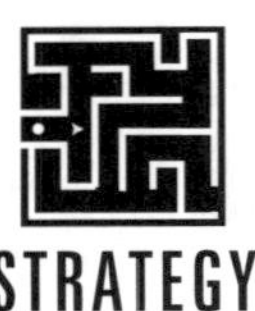
STRATEGY

If a question asks how a certain molecule (e.g., coordination complex, reactant) functions in a given reaction, the answer may use these terms.

20 ACID-BASE CHEMISTRY

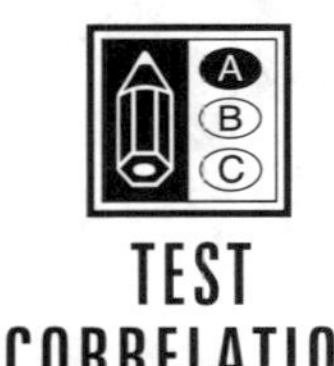

TEST CORRELATION

On the physical sciences section of the MCAT, you may get a passage about physiological buffers in your body. The major physiological buffer of blood is bicarbonate (HCO_3^-), which maintains blood pH at its normal level of 7.4. You must know how buffers act, how to interpret a titration curve involving a buffer, and how to use the Henderson-Hasselbalch equation.

a. Henderson-Hasselbalch equation

$$pH = pK_a + \log\left(\frac{[A^-]}{[HA]}\right)$$

$$pOH = pK_b + \log\left(\frac{[BH^+]}{[B]}\right)$$

$pK_a = -\log(K_a)$
$pH = -\log([H^+])$
K_a = equilibrium constant of acid dissociation

[HA] = concentration of weak acid (M)
$[A^-]$ = concentration of conjugate base (M)
[B] = concentration of weak base (M)
$[BH^+]$ = concentration of conjugate acid (M)

These equations show that the greater the K_a, the lower the pK_a, and the stronger the acid (the lower the pH).

pH works on a logarithmic scale. For example, there is a 100-fold difference in hydrogen ions between a solution with a pH of 2 and a solution with a pH of 4.

When thinking about K_b and pOH, remember that

$$K_w = K_a \times K_b = 1 \times 10^{-14}$$

and that

$$pOH = 14 - pH$$

b. Strong Acid/Strong Base

A strong acid or base dissociates **completely** in water (i.e., moles of strong acid = moles of H^+).

- The six strong acids are HCl, HBr, HI, H_2SO_4, HNO_3, and $HClO_4$. A strong acid has a large K_a. K_a is not useful for strong acids and bases; theoretically, it would be infinite.
- The strong bases are the metal hydroxides from rows 1 and 2 of the periodic table (alkali and alkali earth metals), including NaOH, KOH, and $Ca(OH)_2$, with the exception of $Mg(OH)_2$, which is a weak base.

c. Titration curves

show the pH as a function of the amount of acid $[H^+]$ or base $[OH^-]$ added.

d. Equivalence point

occurs in a titration when the moles of acid equal the moles of base (i.e., equal numbers of equivalents of the acid/base and the titrant have been combined) [Table 2-6].

In the titration of a weak acid with a strong base, the equivalence point is reached when the moles of weak acid equal the moles of strong base (Figure 2-19). Note that this does not mean that concentrations of H^+ equal moles of OH^- (since you usually titrate a weak acid/base with a strong base/acid—otherwise the equivalence point would always be at a pH of 7).

Take, for example, the addition of NaOH to acetic acid CH_3COOH. At low pH, before the NaOH is added, the majority of the acetic acid is protonated. However, as the NaOH concentration increases, an increasing fraction of acetate

TABLE 2-6. When pH = pK_a or pH = equivalence point

When pH = Equivalence Point	When pH = pK_a
Steepest part of the titration curve	Flattest part of the t tration curve
At this point, there is 100% of one species (either A^- or HA)	At this point, there is 50% A^-, 50% HA
Least buffering capacity at this point of the curve	Greatest buffering capacity at this point of the curve
At this point, moles of acid = moles of base	At this point, $([A^-]/[HA]) = 1$

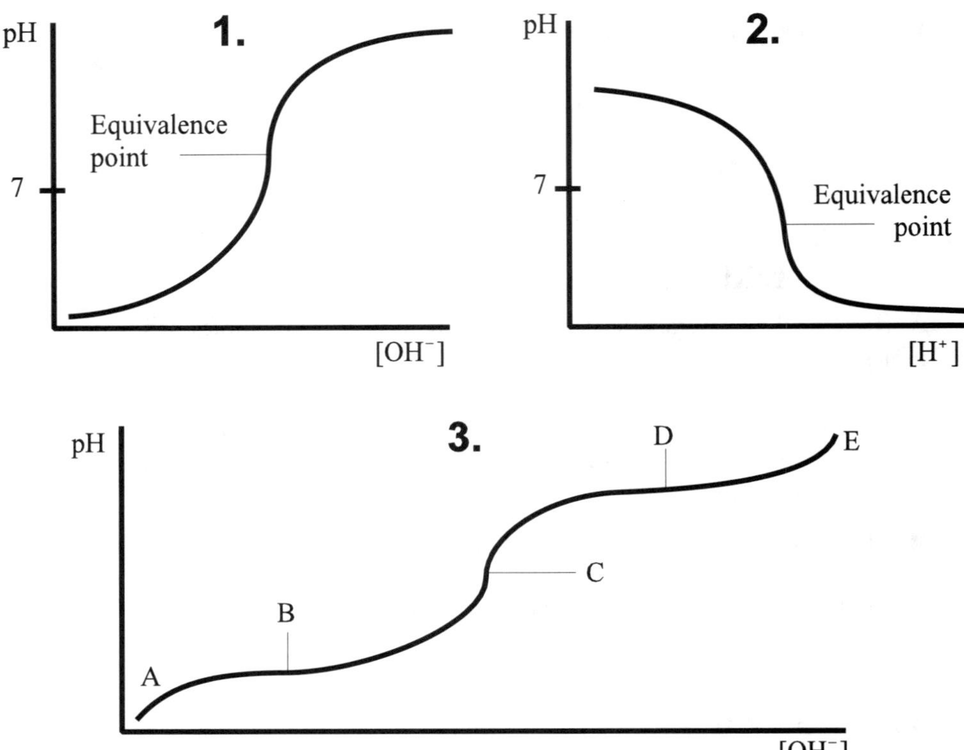

Figure 2-19. Titration of *(1)* a weak acid with a strong base; *(2)* a weak base with a strong acid; and *(3)* a weak diprotic acid with a strong base. *A* = 100% H_2CO_3 (equivalence point #1); *B* = 50% H_2CO_3, 50% HCO_3^- (pH = pK_{a1}); *C* = 100% HCO_3^- (equivalence point #2); *D* = 50% HCO_3^-, 50% CO_3^{2-} (pH = pK_{a2}); *E* = 100% CO_3^{2-} (equivalence point #3).

CH_3COO^- is produced. At the pK_a, the concentration of CH_3COOH is equal to the concentration of CH_3COO^-. For concentrations of OH^- greater than needed to get to the equivalence point, the concentration of CH_3COO^- is greater than the concentration of CH_3COOH.

For a weak acid added to a strong base, the equivalence point is above the neutral pH of 7. For a weak base added to a strong acid, the equivalence point is below the neutral pH of 7. At points B and D, when pH = pK_a, the compound shows the greatest buffering capacity to resist changes in pH (i.e., the flat parts of the titration curve).

F Introduction to the Biological Sciences

Do not get bogged down on any one question or passage.

The last thing you want to see after 3 hours on the verbal reasoning, physical sciences, and essay sections is another section. Then, just when you have had enough, the AAMC hits you with the biological sciences section. Like the physical sciences section, this section has 77 questions to be completed in 100 minutes. Once again, you want to spend 1.25 minutes per question (which leaves you a little extra time for answering hard questions and for checking your answers). Do not get bogged down on any one question or passage; if a particular passage gives you a lot of trouble, skip it and return to it at the end. You can use "batch fill-in" on the answer sheets, but never go to the next passage without filling in the answers from the previous one. The MCAT does not have a penalty for guessing, so answer all questions.

The biggest non–content-related problem that students have with the biological sciences section is fatigue. You begin taking the biological sciences section after hours of previous testing. Most college students have experience with 3- or 4-hour tests, but few have experienced an all-day affair like the MCAT.

- During the break between the essay and the biological sciences section, take a walk outside and load up on sugar (e.g., a candy bar, an endurance bar [Power Bar], a Coke, or even one of the carbo-loading sports drinks).
- Be aware that most people catch their "second wind" and experience increased alertness in the middle of the biological sciences section (the "late afternoon recovery"). Once you finish this section, review your work for careless mistakes.

When studying biology, stress the high-yield concepts associated with the endocrine system, physiology, neurobiology, biochemistry, and cell biology.

According to the AAMC, 65% of the biological sciences section tests concepts from biology and only 35% asks about organic chemistry topics. However, students say that the mix has been about 50–50 on recent exams. Given that the majority of premedical students have strong biology backgrounds and that the AAMC grades the MCAT on a curve, you better know your stuff! Most students have taken more than enough biology courses and tests before they take the MCAT. However, your success on this section does not depend on knowledge of advanced biology. Whereas courses in upper-division biology help you in medical school, much of the advanced biology does not help on the biological sciences section of the MCAT (with the exception of physiology and biochemistry). Instead, you should master the basic biological concepts and processes. Do **not** get lost relearning all the details from all your biology classes. For example, you should master the reactants, products, location, and purpose of glycolysis and the Krebs cycle, but you do not need to memorize all of the intermediate steps.

Organic chemistry is often the premedical student's worst nightmare. It is curious that medical school requires two semesters of organic chemistry. Is it inertia from some 50 years ago, when the biochemical pathways were first discovered? More cynically, is it because admissions committees want to see how you fare under the pressure of blind memorization for no apparent purpose? **The MCAT, however, has been revamped, and the organic chemistry tested on the MCAT is mostly passage-based and all multiple choice. You do not need to memorize every reaction, reagent, and mechanism all over again.** Instead, focus your preparation on reviewing the important concepts of organic chemistry, such as S_N1/E_1 S_N2/E_2 reactions, Markovnikov/anti-Markovnikov addition, and the structures and physical/chemical properties of the different functional groups. Often, the important reactions surface in the passage. In addition, review the different organic chemistry laboratory procedures, such as separation, recrystallization, nuclear magnetic resonance (NMR), infrared (IR) spectroscopy, and chromatography.

Although the test writers state that organic chemistry makes up only 35% of the biological sciences section of the MCAT, many students who have recently taken the exam agree that the split between organic chemistry and biology in the biological sciences section is 50–50.

Know important concepts such as S_N1/S_N2 substitution and Grignard reactions; if you **understand** these reactions, you will be able to deduce the answers to more difficult reaction-based questions presented on the actual exam. Most important, **don't sweat it.** Everyone hates this section, and you need not know most of the brutal details of organic chemistry to do well on the MCAT.

G Organic Chemistry

1 IUPAC NOMENCLATURE AND FUNCTIONAL GROUPS

a. International Union of Pure and Applied Chemistry (IUPAC) Nomenclature

The rules of naming molecules follow this international convention system (Table 2-7). You probably already know that organic chemistry has its own numbering system.

TABLE 2-7. Organic nomenclature for number

Number	Prefix	Number	Prefix
1	meth- (form-)	**6**	hex-
2	eth- (acet-)	**7**	hept-
3	prop-	**8**	oct-
4	but-	**9**	non-
5	pent-	**10**	dec-

b. Functional Groups

In addition, you need to know the **functional groups** in order to name the organic molecules. Functional groups make a molecule distinctive by changing its properties and reactivity. Table 2-8 shows the most important groups to know.

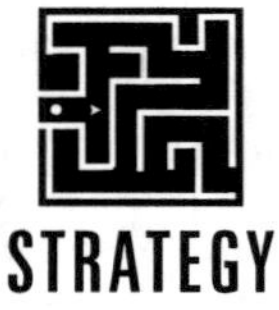

STRATEGY

Use the process of elimination to determine the name of a compound.

Check the multiple-choice answers if you are confused. Start by eliminating answers with the wrong prefix or suffix; then choose from what remains.

- When a molecule has more than one chain or functional group, always name the longest chain first. In addition, assign side chains by the lowest number possible. Often two answers to a question will make sense, but only one follows this IUPAC convention.
- Many common molecules have other common non-IUPAC names, such as acetone (IUPAC name is propanone) or formic acid (methanoic acid). For purposes of the MCAT, know the IUPAC nomenclature system, not these common names; they may appear in a passage, but in most cases the test gives the modern name for the molecule.

TABLE 2-8. Common functional groups

Name	Group	Suffix	Properties	Example
Alkanes	R-CH_2-R	"ane"	1. Formula of C_nH_{2n+2} 2. Nonpolar 3. Boiling and melting points rise with number of carbons, but they decrease with branching 4. All alkanes > 3 carbons have more than one isomer	CH_4 methane
Alkenes	R-CH=CH-R	"ene"	Similar to alkanes—formula of C_nH_{2n}	C_3H_6 propene
Alkynes	R-C≡C-R	"yne"	Similar to alkanes and alkenes—formula of C_nH_{2n-2}. The C≡C bond is shorter and stronger than C−C or C=C.	C_4H_6 butyne
Aromatic Rings	Ph-R	"benzene" "phenyl-"	1. Very stable (Kekulé's ring) 2. Bonds intermediate in length and strength between single and double bonds (hybrid bonds due to resonance)	C_6H_6 benzene C_7H_8 methyl benzene, or toluene
Alcohols	R-OH	"ol"	1. High boiling points due to hydrogen bonding 2. Excellent solutes; dissolve readily in water (polar) 3. Excellent protic solvents due to hydrogen bonding	C_2H_5OH ethanol
Carboxylic Acids	R-COOH	"oic acid"	1. Not as strong as inorganic acids (e.g., HCl); soluble in aqueous base 2. Polar: can form hydrogen bonds 3. Acids with four or fewer carbons are soluble in water; the rest are insoluble 4. Very high boiling points; higher than corresponding alcohols	CH_3-COOH ethanoic acid
Esters	R-COOR	"ate"	1. Polar: can form hydrogen bonds 2. Characteristic odors (like flowers) 3. Larger esters are insoluble in water but soluble in nonpolar organic solvents	C_2H_5-COO-CH_3 methyl propanoate
Ethers	R-O-R	"ether"	1. Very weak polarity 2. Relatively insoluble in water 3. Excellent organic solvents	C_2H_5-O-C_2H_5 diethyl ether
Aldehydes	R-CHO	"aldehyde"	1. Polar compounds 2. High boiling points (lower than alcohols) 3. Capable of hydrogen bonding (acceptor) 4. Only smaller aldehydes are soluble in water	CH_2O formaldehyde
Ketones	R-CO-R	"one"	Similar to aldehydes	CH_3-CO-CH_3 propanone (acetone)
Amines	R-NH_2 R-NH-R′ R-N-R′R″	"amine"	1. Polar—form hydrogen bonds 2. Soluble in water or organic solvents 3. Soluble in dilute acid	CH_3-NH-CH_3 Dimethyl amine

Using the numeric prefixes and functional group suffixes, you should be able to name any compound given on the examination.

HIGH-YIELD FACTS

Give the proper IUPAC nomenclature for the following compounds:

(1) Br Br Cl

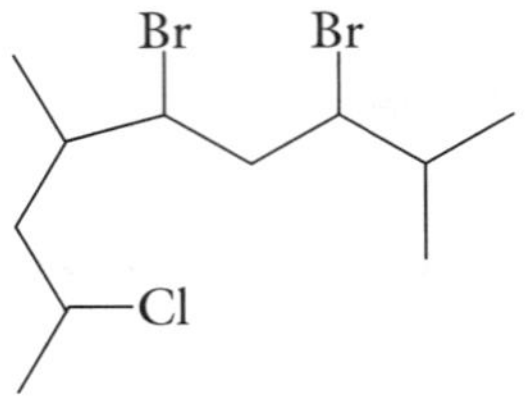

(2) Cl O OH

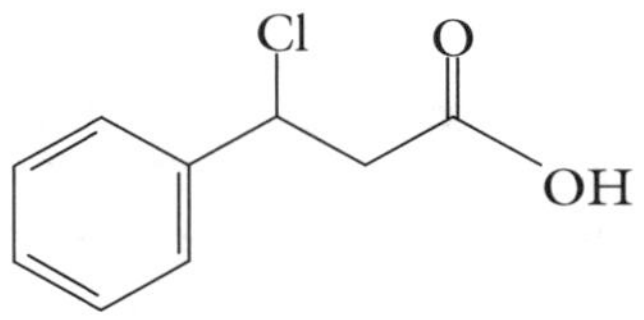

(3) OH

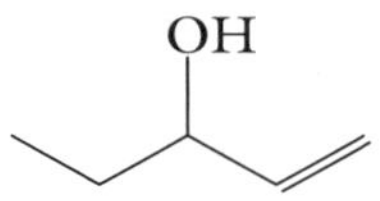

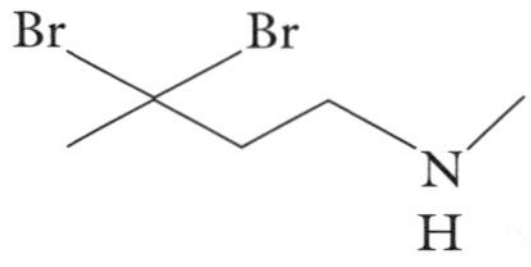

(4) Cl O

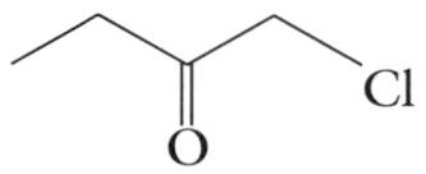

(5) Br Br N H

(1) 3,5-dibromo-8-chloro-2,6-dimethylnonane

(2) 3-chloro-3-phenylpropanoic acid (Remember: The carboxyl group carbon is the lowest numbered carbon)

(3) 1-penten-3-ol

(4) 1-chloro-2-butanone

(5) N-methyl-3,3-dibromo-1-butanamine

Use molecular models to review stereochemistry.

2 STEREOCHEMISTRY

a. Definition

Isomers are different compounds with the same molecular formulas. These compounds often have different physical properties and react differently with the same reagents.

b. Types

The several types of isomers are described next.

1. **Structural isomers** have the same molecular formula but differ in the connectivity of their atoms. The classic examples of structural isomers, the basic type of isomer, are ethyl alcohol (CH_3CH_2OH) and dimethyl ether (CH_3OCH_3). Both have the molecular formula C_2H_6O, but each has different physical and chemical properties (e.g., melting points, boiling points, solubility) and different chemical reactivity because of their different functional groups. The first three alkanes (methane, ethane, and propane) have no structural isomers. Butane has two such isomers:

$CH_3-CH_2-CH_2-CH_3$

Butane (C_4H_{10})

CH_3 / CH_3 — $CH-CH_3$

Isobutane (C_4H_{10})

All alkanes with more than three carbons have at least two structural isomers, and the number of isomers increases with more carbons (e.g., decane has 75 structural isomeric forms). Don't worry about memorizing isomers; just know what a structural isomer is and how to identify two isomers versus two identical structures written differently.

2. **Stereoisomers** do not differ in the connectivity of their atoms but have a different arrangement of atoms in space, for example:

[mirror]

3 CH_3; 1 $BrCH_2$; H 4; 2 C_2H_5 — 4 H; CH_2Br 1; 3 CH_3; 2 C_2H_5

[R]-1-bromo-2-methylbutane [S]-1-bromo-2-methylbutane

3. **Geometric isomers (*cis/trans*, or Z/E, isomers)** differ in the spatial arrangement of atoms around a double bond. When these isomers have two similar chemical groups connected to the central atoms, they can be named via the *cis* (same side) or *trans* (opposite side) nomenclature:

cis-1,2 dichloroethene *trans*-1,2 dichloroethene

When all of the chemical groups connected at the central atoms are different, however, the Z/E nomenclature system must be used. The Z/E nomenclature uses the priority system to classify the attached groups. Generally, the attached atom with the higher atomic weight is assigned the higher priority (e.g., Br has a higher priority than Cl, which in turn has a higher priority than the carbon atom in CH_3). If the two highest priority groups are on the same side of the double bond, a Z isomer is present. In an E isomer, molecules with the two highest priority groups are on different sides of the double bond.

(Z)-1-chloro-2-bromopropene	(E)-1-chloro-2-bromopropene
two high-priority groups (Cl, Br) on **same** side of the double bond	two high-priority groups (Cl, Br) on **different** sides of the double bond

4. **Optical isomers** have chiral centers, which means that the central atom has four different groups attached to it (i.e., it lacks a plane of symmetry). The three types of optical isomers are **enantiomers, diastereomers, and meso compounds.**

5. **Enantiomers (R/S isomers)** are **nonsuperimposable mirror images** of one another. Compounds must have at least one asymmetric or **chiral** carbon to have a pair of enantiomers. Such a carbon must lack a plane of symmetry; that is, if a carbon has two identical substituents (such as two hydrogen atoms), it is not a chiral carbon.

   Enantiomers are named using the R/S system. The groups surrounding a carbon are ranked with the largest group (oxygen, nitrogen) given the highest priority, the second largest group (nitrogen, carbon) given second priority, the next largest group given third priority, and the smallest group (hydrogen) given the lowest priority. Note that you need four different substituent groups on the same carbon to use this method (this is the definition of chirality). Position the molecule so that the lowest ranked group is in the back, and rotate your hand from the highest ranked group to the next-highest ranked group.

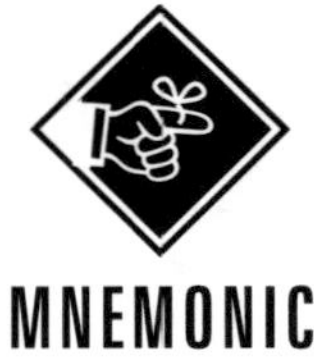

MNEMONIC

If your hand moves clockwise (as if you were making a right turn with a car), you call the carbon an R carbon. If you turn your hand left, it is an S carbon (R = "right turn").

[mirror]

[S]-1-bromo-1-chloroethane	[R]-1-bromo-1-chloroethane

Enantiomers do not differ from one another in most physical or chemical properties, but they do differ in optical activity. One enantiomer will rotate plane-polarized light clockwise (the *d* isomer), and the other will rotate plane-polarized light counterclockwise (*l* isomer).

Optical activity is calculated using the following formula:

$$\alpha_{sp} = \frac{\alpha_{obs}}{cl}$$

α_{sp} = specific rotation of the compound
l = path length (dm)
c = concentration (g/ml)
α_{obs} = experimentally observed rotation

Stereochemistry and the direction of rotation have no known relationship. You cannot predict which enantiomer rotates the light to the right (**dextrorotatory, *d***) and which rotates it to the left (**levorotatory, *l***).

Enantiomeric pairs are hard to separate. A mixture of equal amounts of the two enantiomers is called a **racemic mixture.** Since a racemic mixture contains exactly 50% *d* isomers and 50% *l* isomers, the individual isomer's rotation of polarized light cancels out. Therefore, racemic mixtures do not rotate polarized light (i.e., they are optically inactive).

6. **Diastereomers** are stereoisomers that are not enantiomers (non–mirror-image isomers). They differ in the arrangement of atoms in space but are not mirror images.

Chiral diastereomers are isomers that result from chiral carbons but are not enantiomers. They require **at least two chiral carbons.**

Cl
F C H
C
Br H
CH_3

[1R,2S]-1-chloro-1-fluoro-2-bromopropane

Cl
H C F
C
Br H
CH_3

[1S,2S]-1-chloro-1-fluoro-2-bromopropane

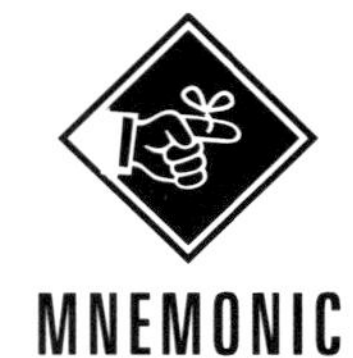

MNEMONIC

Diastereomer: At least two chiral carbons

7. **Meso compounds** are achiral but have asymmetric carbons. They reduce the number of stereoisomers from 2^n (where n is the number of chiral carbons). Although each carbon is asymmetric, the molecule as a whole has a plane of symmetry.

Cl Cl
H—C——C—H
CH_3 CH_3
Plane of symmetry

meso-2,3-dichlorobutane

8. **Conformational (rotational) isomers** differ from each other only by rotation around a carbon–carbon single bond. The molecule can rapidly switch from one rotational isomer to another and thus can usually arrive at the most stable rotational isomer (Figure 2-20). Normally the three conformations are

   - **Anti,** which is the most stable arrangement
   - **Gauche,** which is less stable (a H-CH_3 gauche interaction is more stable than a CH_3-CH_3 interaction)
   - **Eclipsed,** which is the least stable arrangement

Another example of a conformational isomer pair is the chair (most stable—all bonds are in the anti-conformation) versus the boat (less stable—not all bonds are in the anti-conformation) form of cyclohexane. The chair form of cyclohexane minimizes the angle strain, torsional strain, and nonbonded strain of the molecule. Remember that on the cyclohexane molecule, the most stable conformation occurs when the bulky groups occupy the equatorial positions.

Figure 2-20. Internal rotation of 2-methylbutane. Note the three conformations: *anti*—methyl groups are: ±180° rotation—is the most stable (the methyl groups are furthest apart); *gauche*—±60° apart rotation—is less stable than anti; *eclipsed*—0°, ±120° apart rotation—is the least stable arrangement (the most steric interaction).

Give the proper IUPAC nomenclature for the following compounds:

(1) Cl / C_2H_5—C—H / Br

(2)

(3) Br / Cl (structure)

(4) H, Br—C—CH_3, C_2H_5—C—H, Cl (structure)

(5) C_2H_5, Cl—C—CH_3, Cl—C—CH_3, C_2H_5 (structure)

(1) (R)-1-bromo-1-chloropropane

(2) Cis-2-hexene

(3) (E)-2-bromo-3-chloro-2-pentene

(4) (2S,3R)-2-bromo-3-chloropentane

(5) Meso-3,4-dichloro-3,4-dimethyl hexane

3 STABILITY, PHYSICAL PROPERTIES, AND REACTIVITY

The energetic stability of molecules depends on their type of branching, their cis/trans configuration, and the presence of electron-donating or electron-withdrawing groups.

a. Branching

increases the stability of hydrocarbons and the intermolecular repulsion because of increased van der Waals forces, therefore decreasing their boiling point. For example, the branched molecule 2-methylbutene:

$$(CH_3)(H)C{=}C(CH_3)(CH_3)$$

will have a lower boiling point than CH_2=CH-CH_2-CH_2-CH_3 (n-pentene), even though both have the same molecular formula (C_5H_{10}).

Increased stability of molecular compounds is associated with a reduction in the boiling point of the compound. In addition, boiling point is largely dependent on intermolecular forces (e.g., hydrogen bonding).

Cis isomers have higher boiling points than trans isomers because of a net dipole that exists in cis isomers, creating stronger intermolecular forces. Trans isomers have higher melting points because they can stack tighter in a solid matrix than their cis counterpart.

b. *Cis/trans* isomers

like *cis*-2-butene and *trans*-2-butene differ in stability:

$$\underset{cis\text{-2-butene}}{\overset{CH_3\quad\quad CH_3}{C=C}}\qquad \underset{trans\text{-2-butene}}{C=C}$$

cis-2-butene: $CH_3(H)C=C(H)CH_3$ (both CH_3 on the same side)

trans-2-butene: $CH_3(H)C=C(CH_3)H$ (the CH_3 groups on opposite sides)

The *trans* isomer will be more stable than the *cis* isomer because the methyl groups are further apart in the *trans* conformation. This separation leads to less steric interaction and thus to a thermodynamically favored conformation.

Note that the molecule cannot rotate from one form to another because a double bond cannot rotate; therefore, this isomer relationship is different from gauche–anti stability. The *cis* form can exist and will not convert unless the double bond is broken and then reformed.

c. Electron-donating and electron-withdrawing groups

also affect the stability of organic molecules.

According to the Lewis definition, acids are compounds that accept electrons. An electron-withdrawing group makes an organic compound more suitable for accepting electrons and therefore more acidic.

- **Effects on acidic compounds and their conjugate bases**

  Electron-donating groups destabilize the conjugate bases of acidic compounds and decrease the acidity of the compound. Once the acid loses a proton, it has an excess of electrons. Examples of electron-donating groups are OH, NH_2, and OR.

  Electron-withdrawing groups stabilize conjugate bases and therefore increase the acidity of acidic compounds by helping the compounds share the excess electrons of the conjugate base. Examples of electron-withdrawing groups are CO, COOH, and NO_2.

- **Effects on aromatic stability and substitution**

  Electron-donating groups stabilize additions to a benzene ring and increase the reaction rate of electrophilic aromatic substitution. They direct additional substitution to the ortho and para sites. Note that the halogens, which decrease the reaction rate but still direct ortho and para substitution, are an exception to this rule.

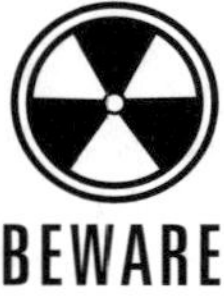
BEWARE

Electron-withdrawing groups decrease the rate of electrophilic aromatic substitution and direct the substitution to the meta site.

4 SUBSTITUTION/ELIMINATION REACTIONS

a. Substitution Reactions of Alkyl Halides

Table 2-9 describes how different types of alkyl halides (primary, secondary, and tertiary) undergo substitution/elimination reactions.

TABLE 2-9. Substitution/elimination reactions of alkyl halides

Reacting Molecule	S_N1	E_1	S_N2	E_2
Primary alkyl halide	Does not react because it cannot form a sufficiently stable carbocation	Does not react because it cannot form stable carbocation	Reacts readily and quickly, fastest in polar aprotic solvent with strong unhindered nucleophile	Reacts favorably with strong, sterically hindered base (e.g., t-butoxide)
Secondary alkyl halide	Reacts slowly if it has an excellent leaving group in a polar protic solvent (E_1 also occurs)	Reacts with good leaving group, in polar protic solvent (enhanced in basic solution)	Reacts only with strong nucleophile (which is not too bulky/branched) in a polar aprotic solvent	Reacts with strong sterically hindered base
Tertiary alkyl halide	Reacts readily (not that quickly) in a polar (nucleophilic) protic solvent	Reacts in non-nucleophilic protic solvent and is enhanced in basic solution	Does not react (steric hindrance)	Reacts somewhat in presence of a strong base

These four reactions have two categories:

1. **Nucleophilic substitution (S_N)**. In this reaction, an incoming nucleophile uses a pair of electrons to form a new carbon bond while displacing the leaving group. This reaction is also called nucleophilic displacement reaction.
2. **Elimination (E).** This reaction occurs when two elements leave a molecule to form a pi bond, thereby changing a carbon–carbon single bond into a carbon–carbon double bond.
3. S_N2 and E_2 are second-order reactions in that two different molecules are involved in their rate-limiting step. The **rate of the reaction, therefore, depends on the concentration of the nucleophile:**

$$\text{rate of } S_N2 \text{ or } E_2 = k\,(\text{electrophile})(\text{nucleophile})$$

4. On the other hand, the S_{N1} and E_1 are first-order reactions, in that the rate-limiting step involves one molecule. The **rate of these reactions is independent of the concentration of the nucleophile.**

$$\text{rate of } S_N1 \text{ or } E_1 = k\,(\text{electrophile})$$

b. S_N2 Reaction

In this one-step reaction, a nucleophile attacks an electrophile while a leaving group simultaneously leaves. This reaction is often called **backside displacement** (Figure 2-21).

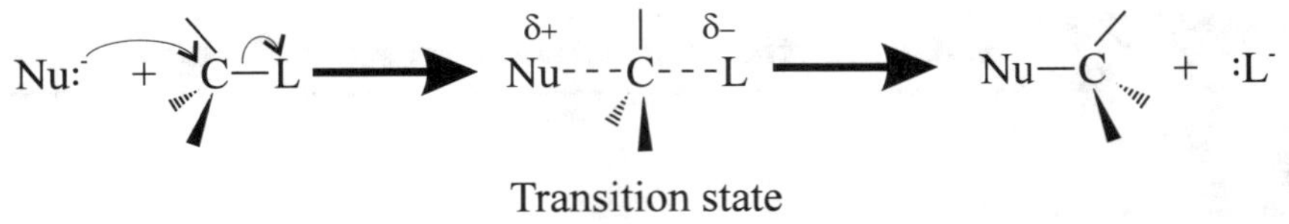

Figure 2-21.
S_N2 reaction: backside displacement.

- The reaction depends on the presence of a strong nucleophile and a good leaving group.
- The stereochemistry of the molecule **inverts** (i.e., R turns to S, and vice versa).
- This reaction is **highly dependent on steric interaction,** which means that primary alkyl halides react best, whereas tertiary alkyl halides barely react at all. Small nucleophiles (e.g., OH) work better than bulky nucleophiles.
- S_N2 works best in **polar aprotic solvents** [e.g., dimethyl sulfoxide (DMSO), N,N-dimethylformamide (DMF)].
- Poor leaving groups (such as OH^-) can be enhanced by compounds such as TsCl (the tosyl group bonds with the O to form a better leaving group).

c. E_2 Reaction

Although similar to S_N2 in that a strong nucleophile attacks an electrophile with a good leaving group, in this reaction, the nucleophile acts as a base and takes a proton from the electrophile, which leads to β **elimination** of the leaving group and the formation of a carbon–carbon double bond (Figure 2-22).

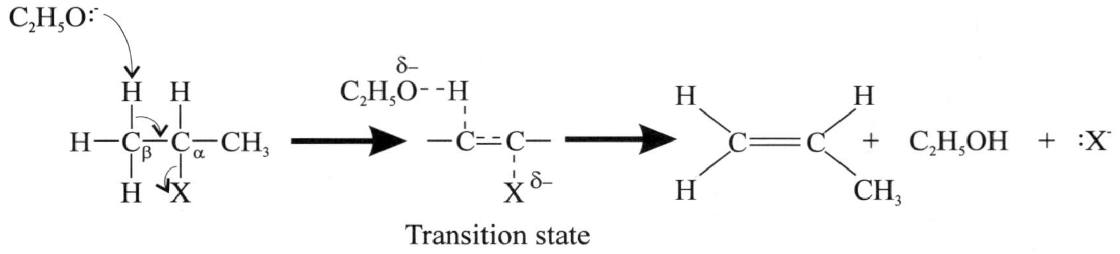

Figure 2-22.
E_2 reaction.

- This reaction is favored over S_N2 if the nucleophile or electrophile is bulky or sterically hindered. E_2 occurs most often when the nucleophile is an especially **strong, bulky base** (e.g, t-butoxide).

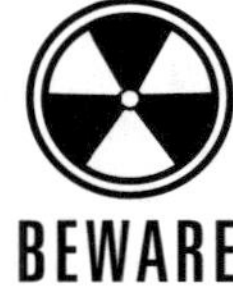

d. S_N1 reaction

is a two-step reaction (Figure 2-23). First, the leaving group is pulled away, forming a carbocation, the rate-limiting step of the reaction. Then, the carbocation is attacked by the nucleophile. Carbocation rearrangement can occur.

- **Stereochemistry is not inverted.** The formation of the carbocation leads to **racemization** because the nucleophile can attack from either side of the carbon, leading to a product that does not rotate polarized light.
- In the first step, loss of the leaving group, the solvent molecule takes part in a **solvolysis** reaction, which works best with **polar protic solvents** (such as formic acid). Polar protic solvents facilitate the solvolysis reaction, leading to the formation of a carbocation intermediate, the rate-determining step.
- This reaction is also improved with tertiary halide electrophiles, which can stabilize the formation of the carbocation.

The formation of the carbocation is the rate-limiting step.

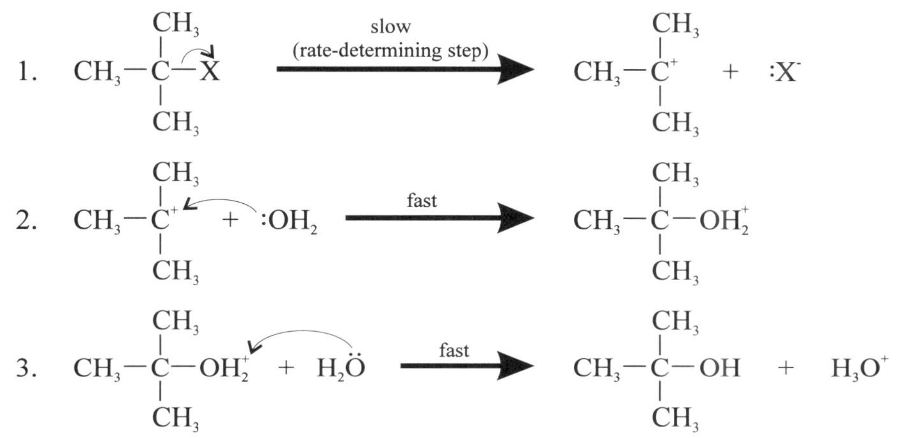

$$1.\quad CH_3{-}C(CH_3)_2{-}X \xrightarrow[\text{(rate-determining step)}]{\text{slow}} CH_3{-}C^+(CH_3)_2 + :X^-$$

$$2.\quad CH_3{-}C^+(CH_3)_2 + :OH_2 \xrightarrow{\text{fast}} CH_3{-}C(CH_3)_2{-}OH_2^+$$

$$3.\quad CH_3{-}C(CH_3)_2{-}OH_2^+ + H_2\ddot{O} \xrightarrow{\text{fast}} CH_3{-}C(CH_3)_2{-}OH + H_3O^+$$

Figure 2-23.
S_N1 reaction.

e. E_1 Reaction

is a two-step alternative to SN1 reaction (Figure 2-24). After the leaving group leaves, the nucleophile picks off a β proton and forms a carbon–carbon double bond. The reaction is favored under circumstances similar to those that favor S_N1: polar protic solvents and tertiary halides.

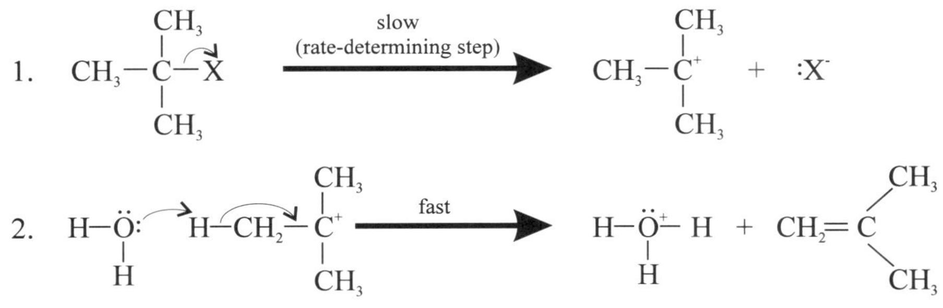

$$1.\quad CH_3{-}C(CH_3)_2{-}X \xrightarrow[\text{(rate-determining step)}]{\text{slow}} CH_3{-}C^+(CH_3)_2 + :X^-$$

$$2.\quad H{-}\ddot{O}(H){:}\ \ H{-}CH_2{-}C^+(CH_3)_2 \xrightarrow{\text{fast}} H{-}\ddot{O}^+(H){-}H + CH_2{=}C(CH_3)_2$$

Figure 2-24.
E_1 reaction.

High temperatures favor elimination reactions. If the MCAT sketches a reaction with heat (Δ) as one reactant, but you don't know the product, the best answer choice is the one in which the molecule formed has a double bond.

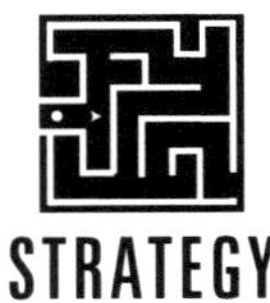
STRATEGY

QUESTION

All of the following statements about organic substitution and elimination reactions are true EXCEPT:

(a) The rate of an S_N1/E_1 reaction does not depend on the concentration of the nucleophile.

(b) S_N2 reactions are favored by the use of polar aprotic solvents (e.g., DMSO, DMF).

(c) S_N2 reactions result in a product that is a racemic mixture and optically inactive.

(d) E_2 reactions are favored by high temperatures and the use of a strong, bulky base (e.g., t-butoxide).

ANSWER

The answer is **c.** Because S_N2 reactions are one-step reactions in which a nucleophile attacks an electrophile while a leaving group is simultaneously displaced, this results in a backside displacement that causes the stereochemistry of the molecule to invert. S_N1 reactions result in a product that is a racemic mixture and optically inactive through the formation of a carbocation intermediate, which is the rate-determining step of the reaction.

5 MARKOVNIKOV'S RULE AND ITS EXCEPTIONS

a. Markovnikov's rule

Whenever a molecule H−X (X is a halogen) is added to an alkene, the halogen bonds to the more substituted carbon and the hydrogen bonds to the less substituted carbon.

1. The guiding principle for this reaction is that **the more stable carbocation must be formed,** which happens when the positive charge of the carbocation is on the more substituted carbon. The halogen thus attacks the more substituted carbon, as Markovnikov's rule predicts.

2. The other important feature of the Markovnikov reaction is the chronology of the mechanism: **the carbocation forms first** as the proton bonds with the less substituted carbon; then the halogen anion bonds to the positively charged (more substituted) carbon. This chronology is important because the stability of the carbocation affects the specific formation of the product.

b. The basic concepts

behind this law affect the selectivity/regiochemistry of many other organic reactions. An example of Markovnikov addition follows:

$$(CH_3)_2C{=}CH_2 \xrightarrow[\text{Markovnikov addition}]{HBr} (CH_3)_2CBrCH_3 \text{ Major product}$$

$$(CH_3)_2C{=}CH_2 \xrightarrow[\text{Anti-Markovnikov addition}]{HBr,\ \textbf{Peroxides (ROOR')}} (CH_3)_2CHCH_2Br \text{ Major product}$$

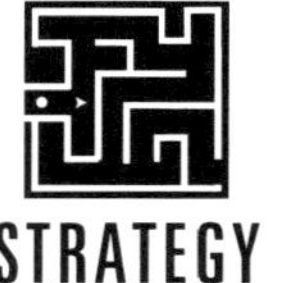
STRATEGY

c. Exceptions

Not all H−X addition reactions happen according to Markovnikov's rule, however; this rule merely describes the thermodynamically favored reaction (i.e., the reaction that occurs in the absence of large amounts of energy or in the absence of a catalyst). Peroxides are excellent catalysts of anti-Markovnikov addition reactions.

The same principle applies to other addition reactions involving alkenes, such as the addition of H_2O to an alkene to form an alcohol. Under normal conditions (high temperatures, hydrating environment), the addition of H_2O to an alkene in the presence of an acid will form a Markovnikov alcohol so that the OH group is on the more substituted carbon. However, using a process called **hydroboration** (B_2H_6), an alcohol can be formed from an alkene so that the OH goes to the less substituted carbon (anti-Markovnikov addition).

6 GRIGNARD REACTIONS

a. Definition

A Grignard reaction yields a compound with a carbon–magnesium bond; the carbon bonded to this magnesium can then act as a nucleophile and form a carbon–carbon bond with any electrophilic carbon.

Chemical industries use **Grignard reactions to synthesize carbon–carbon bonds,** which prove to be very useful in a variety of organic reactions. In some cases, organolithium reagents can be used in place of Grignard reagents.

1. A Grignard reagent can be formed by mixing an alkyl halide with magnesium, stirring in an ether solvent (a popular lab question on the MCAT):

$$CH_3{-}CH_2{-}CH_2{-}Br + Mg \xrightarrow{(C_2H_5)_2O} CH_3{-}CH_2{-}CH_2{-}Mg{-}Br$$

(propylmagnesium bromide)

Because of its carbon–metal bond, a Grignard reagent is an organometallic compound.

2. The most common Grignard reaction is the synthesis of alcohols from aldehydes and ketones:

$$>C{=}O + R{-}Mg{-}X \xrightarrow{(C_2H_5)_2O} -\underset{R}{\overset{|}{C}}-O^-Mg^+X \xrightarrow{H_2O} -\underset{R}{\overset{|}{C}}-OH$$

This reaction is simple. The R group acts as a nucleophile and attacks the carbon, which causes the oxygen to form a bond with the MgX portion of the Grignard reaction. The final step is an "H_2O wash," which cleaves the O–MgX bond and leaves the hydrocarbon in its alcohol form.

3. The other Grignard reactions roughly follow the model of the preparation of alcohols. For the MCAT, just remember and understand the preceding reaction and apply it to questions about other Grignard reactions.

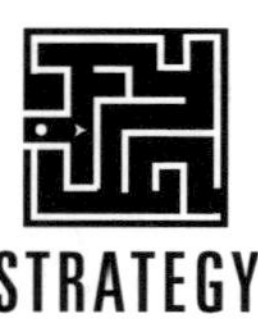
STRATEGY

b. One other Grignard reaction

that is worth committing to memory is the formation of carboxylic acids by bubbling gaseous CO_2 into an ether solution of the Grignard reagent or by pouring the Grignard reagent over dry ice.

QUESTION

Provide the structure as well as the IUPAC name of the missing products/intermediates in the following multi-step reactions:

$$\text{(a)}\ CH_3Br \xrightarrow[Et_2O]{Mg} \xrightarrow[H_2O]{\text{ethylene oxide } (CH_2CH_2O)} \xrightarrow{PBr_3} \xrightarrow[Et_2O]{Mg} \xrightarrow[H_2O]{} \boxed{?}$$

(b) [?] $\xrightarrow[Et_2O]{Mg}$ $\xrightarrow[H_2O]{CH_3CH_2C(=O)CH_3}$ $\xrightarrow{PBr_3}$ $\xrightarrow[Et_2O]{Mg}$ $\xrightarrow{CO_2}$ $(CH_3)_2CHC(CH_3)(CH_2CH_3)COOH$

(c) $CH_3CH_2Br \xrightarrow[Et_2O]{Mg} CH_3CH_2MgBr \xrightarrow[H_2O]{H_2C=O}$ [?] $\xrightarrow{KMnO_4} CH_3CH_2COOH$

(a) $CH_3Br \xrightarrow[Et_2O]{Mg} CH_3MgBr \xrightarrow{CH_2CH_2O\ (\text{ethylene oxide})} CH_3CH_2CH_2OH$

$\xrightarrow{PBr_3} CH_3CH_2CH_2Br \xrightarrow[Et_2O]{Mg} CH_3CH_2CH_2MgBr$

$\xrightarrow[H_2O]{} CH_3CH_2CH_3$ (n-propane)

(b) **Working backward**s:

$(CH_3)_2CHC(CH_3)(CH_2CH_3)COOH \xleftarrow{CO_2} \xleftarrow[Et_2O]{Mg} (CH_3)_2CHC(CH_3)(CH_2CH_3)Br \xleftarrow{PBr_3}$

$(CH_3)_2CHC(CH_3)(CH_2CH_3)OH \xleftarrow[H_2O]{CH_3CH_2C(=O)CH_3} \xleftarrow[Et_2O]{Mg} (CH_3)_2CH{-}Br$

(2-bromopropane)

(c) $CH_3CH_2Br \xrightarrow[Et_2O]{Mg} CH_3CH_2MgBr \xrightarrow[H_2O]{H_2C=O} CH_3CH_2CH_2OH$ (1-propanol)

$\xrightarrow{KMnO_4} CH_3CH_2COOH$

7 OXIDIZING AND REDUCING AGENTS

a. An oxidizing agent

is a chemical compound or mixture of compounds in solution that brings about the oxidation of another compound (i.e., a loss of electrons); the oxidizing agent is in turn reduced (because for each oxidation reaction there must be a reduction reaction). Oxidizing agents increase the number of carbon/oxygen bonds and reduce the number of carbon/hydrogen and hydrogen/oxygen bonds (e.g., the transformation of an alcohol to an aldehyde).

b. A reducing agent

is a chemical compound or mixture of compounds in solution that brings about the reduction of another compound (i.e., a gain of electrons); the reducing agent is in turn oxidized. Reducing agents decrease the number of carbon/oxygen bonds and increase the number of carbon/hydrogen and hydrogen/oxygen bonds (e.g., the transformation of a ketone/aldehyde to an alcohol).

c. Oxidation and reduction reactions

are considered fundamental concepts within organic chemistry (Table 2-10). Many different oxidizing and reducing agents may prove useful for converting one organic compound to another, for example:

$CH_3CH_2OH + KMnO_4 \rightarrow CH_3COOH$ (oxidation of an alcohol to a carboxylic acid)

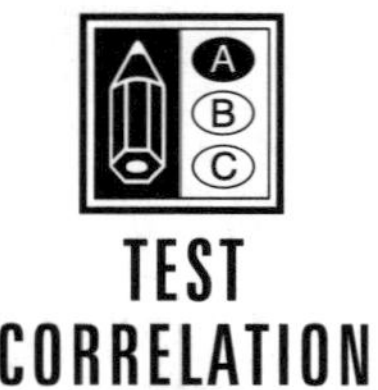

TEST CORRELATION

Oxidation and reduction reactions are very popular reactions on the MCAT; they test your knowledge of the interconversion of various organic chemical functional groups. In addition, the concept of redox appears again and again on the general chemistry section. Therefore, you must be able to identify oxidizing and reducing agents, know how they function in the reaction, and know what products they yield.

TABLE 2-10. Major oxidizing and reducing agents and the reactions/conversions they can direct

Oxidizing Agents	Reactions/Conversions
$KMnO_4$	Primary alcohols → carboxylic acids
Cr_2O_7	Primary alcohols → aldehydes → carboxylic acids
CrO_4	Secondary alcohols → ketones Tertiary alcohols (do not react)
OsO_4	Alkenes → diols
O_3	Alkenes → ketones (ozonolysis)
	Reducing Agents
$LiAlH_4$	Aldehydes → alcohols Ketones → alcohols Carboxylic acids → alcohols
$NaBH_4$	Aldehydes → alcohols Ketones → alcohols (less reactive than $LiAlH_4$)

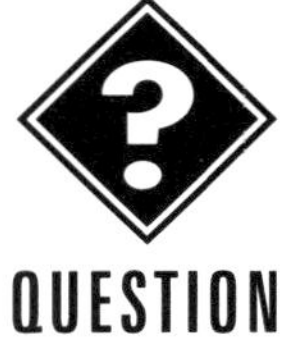

Provide the structure and IUPAC name of the missing products in the following reactions:

(a) $CH_3CH_2OH \xrightarrow{KMnO_4} \boxed{?}$

(b) $(CH_3)_2C{=}CH_2 \xrightarrow[ROOR']{HBr} \xrightarrow[(C_2H_5)_2O]{Mg} \xrightarrow[H_2O]{CO_2} \xrightarrow{LiAlH_4} \boxed{?}$

(c) $(CH_3)_3COH \xrightarrow{CrO_3} \boxed{?}$

(a) Because $KMnO_4$ is a strong oxidizing agent, it will oxidize a primary alcohol into a carboxylic acid:

$$\underset{\text{(ethanol)}}{CH_3CH_2OH} \xrightarrow{KMnO_4} \underset{\text{ethanoic acid (acetic acid)}}{CH_3COOH}$$

(b) Expect to see a few multi-step reactions on the MCAT. The best way to attack this problem is one step at a time:

$$(CH_3)_2C{=}CH_2 \xrightarrow[\text{ROOR' (anti-Markovnikov addition)}]{\text{HBr}} (CH_3)_2CHCH_2Br$$

$$\xrightarrow[\text{Et}_2\text{O (Grignard reagent)}]{\text{Mg}} (CH_3)_2CHCH_2MgBr$$

$$\xrightarrow[H_2O]{CO_2} (CH_3)_2CHCH_2COOH$$

$$\xrightarrow[\text{(reducing agent)}]{LiAlH_4} (CH_3)_2CHCH_2CH_2OH$$

(3-methyl-1-butanol or 3-methylbutanol; isopentanol is the common name, not the IUPAC nomenclature)

(c) Tertiary alcohols cannot be oxidized. Thus, *no reaction* occurs and the product remains 2-methyl-2-propanol (tert-butyl alcohol is the common name, not the IUPAC nomenclature).

8 OTHER ORGANIC REACTIONS

Most other organic reactions are not worth memorizing. Nevertheless, you should review these reactions so you can understand them if they are on the MCAT examination:

- Hydrogenation of alkenes (with Pt as the catalyst)
- Diels-Alder reaction (dienes to cyclic alkenes—just look at it; it's pretty complex)
- Ester synthesis (usually in the presence of a dehydrating agent)
- Friedel–Crafts alkylation/acylation ($AlCl_3$ serves as a Lewis acid to destabilize the aromatic ring)
- Williamson ether synthesis (S_N2 reaction of alkyl halide with alkoxide)

- Ozonolysis
- Three ways of synthesizing a carboxylic acid: Grignard addition of carbon dioxide, oxidation of aldehydes and primary alcohols, and hydrolysis of nitriles (examples of each are found in Section 10 "High-Yield Organic Chemistry Reactions")
- Diazonium salts: Interconversion of functional groups on aromatic rings
- Reactions involving Schiff bases

9 CHEMICAL PURIFICATION

a. Extraction

is the separation of a compound from a solid material by precipitating it out of solution or the separation of components from a liquid mixture using a separatory funnel (when the compound you want does not mix with the solvent of choice).

b. Centrifugation

is separating materials by using a machine that applies a centrifugal force to induce sedimentation.

c. Filtration

is the separation of a solid from a liquid or gas via a membrane that allows the liquid or gas to pass through without the solid.

d. Distillation

is the separation of multiple liquids by boiling off the liquid that has the lower boiling point and then collecting it in a condensation tube.

e. Fractional distillation

is most effective for separating two liquids that have similar boiling points (that differ by a few degrees).

f. Recrystallization

is precipitating a crystal by repeatedly manipulating the temperature of the solution, which removes impurities and purifies the crystal.

g. Sublimation

is the purification of a solid by vaporizing it directly to the gaseous phase. Condense the vapor using a cold finger, which is a piece of glassware with cold water running through it.

h. Electrophoresis

is the separation of proteins or nucleic acids (DNA/RNA) in a gel based on size, net charge, or both (Figure 2-25). Sodium dodecyl sulfate (SDS) electrophoresis separates proteins on the basis of size only. It is useful only for determining the molecular weights of single-subunit proteins, because SDS denatures proteins into single subunits. Migration of denatured compounds on SDS electrophoresis is inversely proportional to the molecular weight of the denatured compound. If the molecular weight of a multiple-subunit protein needs to be determined, then gel filtration can be used.

i. Gel filtration

is the separation of proteins or nucleic acids (DNA/RNA) based on molecular weight. In gel filtration, a glass column is filled with Sephadex beads that contain micropores of a specific diameter. The liquid containing the protein or nucleic acid is run through the column. Water is then used as an eluent. Large molecules exit

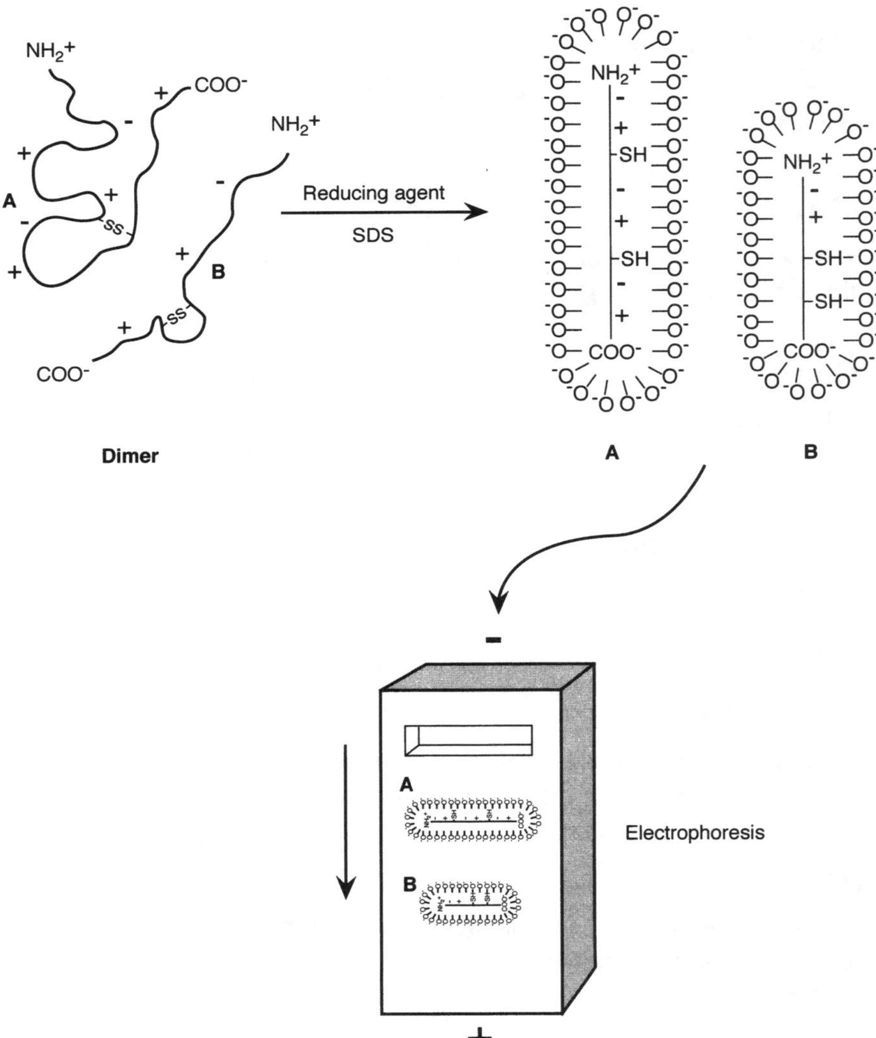

Figure 2-25.
Proteins can be separated on the basis of their size by sodium dodecyl sulfate (SDS) polyacrylamide gel electrophoresis. Proteins are heated with SDS and a reducing agent, which breaks the disulfide bonds. The SDS forms negatively charged micelles around the protein. When these proteins are run through a cross-linked polyacrylamide gel in an electric field, all micelle-proteins move toward the positive pole. The small molecules *(B)* migrate through the gel faster than the large molecules *(A)*. (Reprinted with permission from Davidson VL, Sittman DB: *NMS Biochemistry,* 3rd ed. Baltimore, Williams & Wilkins, 1994, p 40.)

the column first; smaller molecules get stuck in the micropores of the beads, taking more time to elute down the column. Unlike SDS electrophoresis, denaturing agents are not used; therefore, the molecular weights of multiple-subunit proteins can be determined. Gel filtration also can be used to purify proteins (e.g., enzymes, snake venom).

j. Chromatography

is the separation of components based on the strength of their affinity for an adsorbent.

1. **Phases.** Chromatography systems consist of two phases:

   (a) **Stationary phase (adsorbent)** is the foundation onto which the mixture of compounds is loaded. This phase usually consists of a specific type of medium that has specific affinities for various chemical compounds.

   (b) **Mobile phase (eluent)** is usually an organic solvent that moves through the adsorbent at specific rates, depending on the relative polarities of the compound, adsorbent, and eluent.

2. **Types** of chromatography include:

   (a) **Thin-layer chromatography.** The adsorbent is silica gel or aluminum oxide (polar). The eluent is a nonpolar organic solvent (e.g., hexane, benzene). The driving force is capillary action.

   $$\text{Ratio of fronts } (R_f) \text{ value } = \frac{\text{Distance the compound migrated}}{\text{Distance the eluent migrated}}$$

   The R_f value is inversely proportional to the polarity of the compound. Assuming that a relatively nonpolar eluent is used, the higher the compound's R_f value for a specific eluent, the more nonpolar the compound will be. The more nonpolar the eluent is, the lower the R_f value for a specific compound will be, because the more nonpolar eluent is less likely to carry along the polar adsorbent.

   (b) **Column chromatography.** The adsorbent is silica gel or aluminum oxide (polar). The eluent is a nonpolar organic solvent (e.g., hexane, benzene). The driving force is gravity. Similar to thin-layer chromatography, the more nonpolar a compound is, the more rapidly the compound will elute.

   (c) **Gas chromatography.** The adsorbent is a polar-coiled column. The eluent is a nonpolar, chemically inert gas (e.g., hydrogen, nitrogen, or helium). The driving force is vapor pressure. The retention time, which is the time it takes for the specific compound to elute through the column, is measured. The more polar the compound is, the longer retention time it will have.

   (d) **High-performance liquid chromatography.** The adsorbent is a polar-coiled column. The eluent is a nonpolar, organic liquid (e.g., hexane, benzene). The driving force is pressure. Conceptually, high-performance liquid chromatography is similar to gas chromatography.

10 HIGH-YIELD ORGANIC CHEMISTRY REACTIONS

a. Alkanes

1. Preparation

(a) Hydrogenation of Alkenes

$$CH_2{=}CH_2 \xrightarrow[\text{Pt, Pd, or Ni}]{H_2} CH_3CH_3$$

(b) Hydrolysis of a Grignard Reagent

$$CH_3CH_2Br \xrightarrow[Et_2O]{Mg} CH_3CH_2MgBr \xrightarrow{H_2O} CH_3CH_3$$

(c) Reduction of an Alkyl Halide

$$CH_3CH_2CH_2Br \xrightarrow[Zn]{H_2} CH_3CH_2CH_3$$

2. Reactions

Free Radical Halogenation

$$Br_2 \xrightarrow{\text{heat or light}} 2\,Br\cdot \quad \text{[Chain Initiating Step]}$$

$$\left.\begin{array}{l} Br\cdot + CH_3CH_3 \longrightarrow HBr + CH_3CH_2\cdot \\ CH_3CH_2\cdot + Br_2 \longrightarrow CH_3CH_2Br + Br\cdot \end{array}\right] \text{[Chain Propagating Steps]}$$

$$\left.\begin{array}{l} Br\cdot + Br\cdot \longrightarrow Br_2 \\ CH_3CH_2\cdot + CH_3CH_2\cdot \longrightarrow CH_3CH_2CH_2CH_3 \\ CH_3CH_2\cdot + Br\cdot \longrightarrow CH_3CH_2Br \end{array}\right] \text{[Chain Terminating Steps]}$$

b. Alkyl Halides

1. Preparation

(a) Halogenation of Alcohols

$$CH_3CH_2OH \xrightarrow[\text{or HBr}]{PBr_3} CH_3CH_2Br$$

(b) Free Radical Halogenation of Alkanes

$$CH_3CH_3 \xrightarrow[\text{Heat or light}]{Br_2} CH_3CH_2Br + HBr$$

(c) Hydrohalogenation of Alkenes—Markovnikov Addition

$$(CH_3)(CH_3CH_2)C{=}C(H)(CH_3) \xrightarrow{HBr} CH_3CH_2C(CH_3)(Br)CH_2CH_3$$

(d) Addition of Halogens to Alkenes and Alkynes

$$CH_2{=}CH_2 \xrightarrow{Br_2} BrCH_2CH_2Br \text{ (anti-addition)}$$

$$HC{\equiv}CH \xrightarrow{2Br_2} Br_2CHCHBr_2$$

2. Reactions

(a) Substitution Reactions

$$CH_3Br \xrightarrow{NaOH \text{ or } H_2O} CH_3OH$$

$$CH_3Br \xrightarrow{CN^-} CH_3C{\equiv}N$$

$$CH_3Br \xrightarrow{:NH_3} CH_3NH_2$$

(b) Williamson Synthesis of Ethers

$$CH_3Br + {}^-OCH_2CH_3 \longrightarrow CH_3OCH_2CH_3$$

(c) Friedel–Crafts Reaction

$$CH_3CH_2Br \xrightarrow[AlCl_3]{C_6H_6} C_6H_5{-}CH_2CH_3$$

(d) Dehydrohalogenation of Alkenes (E2 Reaction) with a Strong, Bulky Base

$$CH_3CH_2Br \xrightarrow[E_2]{NaOC(CH_3)_3} CH_2{=}CH_2$$

(e) Grignard Reactions

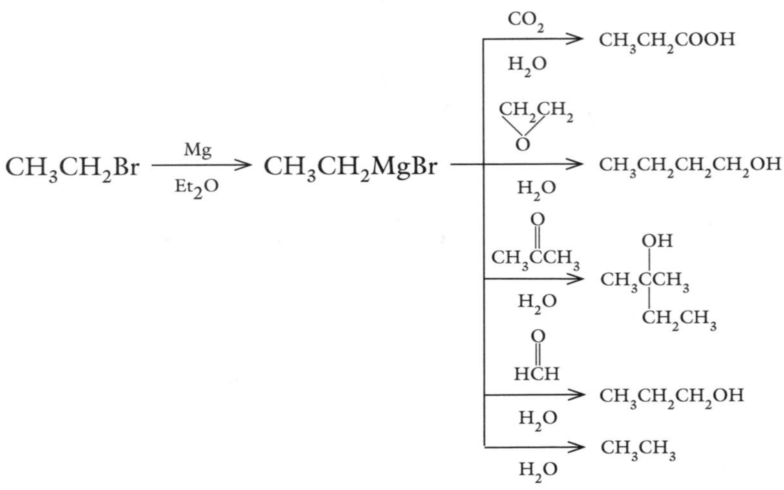

(f) Reduction to an Alkane

$$CH_3CH_2Br \xrightarrow[Zn]{H_2} CH_3CH_3$$

c. Alkenes

1. Preparation

(a) Dehydrohalogenation of Alkyl Halides (E_2 Reaction) with a Strong, Bulky Base

$$CH_3CH_2Br \xrightarrow[E_2]{NaOC(CH_3)_3} CH_2{=}CH_2$$

(b) Dehydration of Alcohols

$$CH_3CH_2CH_2OH \xrightarrow{H^+} CH_3CH{=}CH_2$$

(c) Reduction of Alkynes

$$HC{\equiv}CH \xrightarrow[\text{Lindlar Catalyst}]{H_2} CH_2{=}CH_2 \text{ (syn addition)}$$

2. Reactions

(a) Reduction to Alkanes

$$CH_2{=}CH_2 \xrightarrow[\text{Pt, Pd, or Ni}]{H_2} CH_3CH_3 \text{ (syn addition)}$$

(b) Addition of Halogens

Cyclopentene $\xrightarrow{Br_2}$ trans-1,2-dibromocyclopentane (Br, H / H, Br) (anti-addition)

(c) Hydrohalogenation of Alkenes

$(CH_3)(CH_3CH_2)C{=}CH_2 \xrightarrow{HBr} CH_3CH_2C(CH_3)(Br)CH_3$ (Markovnikov addition)

$(CH_3)(CH_3CH_2)C{=}CH_2 \xrightarrow[\text{ROOR (peroxide)}]{HBr} CH_3CH_2CH(CH_3)CH_2Br$ (anti-Markovnikov addition)

(d) Hydration of Alkenes

$(CH_3)(CH_3CH_2)C{=}CH_2 \xrightarrow[H^+]{H_2O} CH_3CH_2C(OH)(CH_3)CH_3$ (Markovnikov addition)

(e) Halohydrin Formation of Alkenes

-OH Group Adds by Markovnikov Addition

$(CH_3)(CH_3CH_2)C{=}CH_2 \xrightarrow[H_2O]{Br_2} CH_3CH_2C(CH_3)(OH)CH_2Br$

(f) Oxymercuration–Demercuration

$(CH_3)(CH_3CH_2)C{=}CH_2 \xrightarrow[NaBH_4]{Hg(OAc)_2} CH_3CH_2C(CH_3)(OH)CH_3$ (Markovnikov addition)

(g) Hydroboration–Oxidation

$(CH_3)(CH_3CH_2)C{=}CH_2 \xrightarrow[(2)H_2O_2, OH^-]{(1)(BH_3)_2} CH_3CH_2CH(CH_3)CH_2OH$ (Anti-Markovnikov addition)

(h) Ozonolysis Cleavage of Alkanes

$$(CH_3)(CH_3CH_2)C{=}CH_2 \xrightarrow[(2)H_2O,Zn]{(1)O_3} (CH_3)(CH_3CH_2)C{=}O + O{=}CH_2$$

$$\text{cyclohexene} \xrightarrow[(2)H_2O,Zn]{(1)O_3} OHC{-}CH_2CH_2CH_2CH_2{-}CHO$$

d. Alcohols

1. Preparation

(a) Preparation from Alkenes

$$(CH_3)(CH_3CH_2)C{=}CH_2 \xrightarrow[\text{or } Hg(OAc)_2,\ NaBH_4]{H_2O,H^+} CH_3CH_2C(CH_3)(OH)CH_3 \text{ (Markovnikov addition)}$$

$$(CH_3)(CH_3CH_2)C{=}CH_2 \xrightarrow[(2)H_2O_2,\ OH^-]{(1)(BH_3)_2} CH_3CH_2CH(CH_3)CH_2OH \text{ (Anti-Markovnikov addition)}$$

(b) Grignard Synthesis from Alkyl Halides

$$CH_3CH_2Br \xrightarrow[Et_2O]{Mg} CH_3CH_2MgBr$$

$$CH_3CH_2MgBr \xrightarrow[H_2O]{CH_2CH_2O \text{ (ethylene oxide)}} CH_3CH_2CH_2CH_2OH \quad 1^\circ \text{ Alcohols}$$

$$CH_3CH_2MgBr \xrightarrow[H_2O]{HCHO} CH_3CH_2CH_2OH \quad 1^\circ \text{ Alcohols}$$

$$CH_3CH_2MgBr \xrightarrow[H_2O]{CH_3CHO} CH_3CH(OH)CH_2CH_3 \quad 2^\circ \text{ Alcohol}$$

$$CH_3CH_2MgBr \xrightarrow[H_2O]{CH_3COCH_3} CH_3C(OH)(CH_3)CH_2CH_3 \quad 3^\circ \text{ Alcohol}$$

(c) Hydrolysis of Alkyl Halides

$$CH_3CH_2Br \xrightarrow[S_n2]{NaOH} CH_3CH_2OH$$

(d) Reduction of Carboxylic Acids

$$CH_3CH_2COOH \xrightarrow{LiAlH_4} CH_3CH_2CH_2OH$$

2. Reactions

(a) Conversion to Alkyl Halides

$$CH_3CH_2OH \xrightarrow[\text{or conc. HBr}]{PBr_3} CH_3CH_2Br \xrightarrow{CH_3ONa} CH_3CH_2OCH_3$$

(b) Dehydration of Alcohols to Alkenes

$$CH_3CH_2CH_2OH \xrightarrow{H^+} CH_3CH{=}CH_2 + H_2O$$

(c) Esterification (Alcohol + Carboxylic Acid = Ester)

$$CH_3CH_2OH + (CH_3)_2CHCOOH \xrightarrow{H^+} (CH_3)_2CHCOOCH_2CH_3$$

(d) Oxidation

$$CH_3CH_2OH \xrightarrow[\text{or } Cr_2O_7^-]{CrO_3} CH_3\overset{O}{\overset{\|}{C}}H \xrightarrow[\text{or } Cr_2O_7^-]{CrO_3} CH_3COOH$$

$$CH_3CH_2OH \xrightarrow{KMnO_4} CH_3COOH$$

$$(CH_3)_2CHOH \xrightarrow[\text{or } KMnO_4]{CrO_3} CH_3\overset{O}{\overset{\|}{C}}CH_3$$

$$CH_3-\underset{CH_3}{\overset{OH}{C}}-CH_3 \xrightarrow{KMnO_4} \text{No Reaction}$$

(Tertiary alcohols cannot be oxidized.)

(e) Addition of Tosyl Chloride

$$CH_3CH_2OH \xrightarrow{TsCl} CH_3CH_2\underbrace{OTs}_{\text{good leaving group}}$$

$$CH_3CH_2OTs \xrightarrow{OH^-} CH_3CH_2OH$$

$$CH_3CH_2OTs \xrightarrow{I^-} CH_3CH_2I$$

$$CH_3CH_2OTs \xrightarrow{CN^-} CH_3CH_2CN$$

e. Ethers

1. Preparation

(a) Williamson Synthesis of Ethers

$$CH_3CH_2OH \xrightarrow{Na} CH_3CH_2O^- \xrightarrow{CH_3Br} CH_3CH_2OCH_3$$

(b) Alkoxymercuration–Demercuration

$$CH_3CH{=}CH_2 + CH_3CH_2CH_2OH \xrightarrow[NaBH_4]{Hg(OOCCF_3)_2} CH_3CH(OCH_2CH_2CH_3)CH_3$$

(Markovnikov addition)

2. Reactions

Cleavage by Acids

$$CH_3CH_2OCH_3 \xrightarrow{HBr} CH_3CH_2Br + CH_3OH$$

f. Aldehydes and Ketones

1. Preparation

(a) Oxidation of Alcohols

$$CH_3CH_2CH_2OH \xrightarrow{CrO_3} CH_3CH_2CH{=}O$$

$$CH_3CH(OH)CH_3 \xrightarrow{CrO_3} CH_3C({=}O)CH_3$$

(b) Friedel–Crafts Acylation

$$CH_3CH_2C({=}O){-}Cl + C_6H_6 \xrightarrow{AlCl_3} C_6H_5C({=}O)CH_2CH_3$$

(c) Reaction of Acyl Chlorides with Organolithium Reagents

$$CH_3Br \xrightarrow[Et_2O]{Li} CH_3Li \xrightarrow{CuBr} (CH_3)_2CuLi$$

$$\xrightarrow{CH_3CH_2C(=O)Cl} CH_3CH_2C({=}O)CH_3$$

2. Reactions

(a) Oxidation and Reduction

$$CH_3CH_2OH \underset{NaBH_4}{\overset{CrO_3}{\rightleftharpoons}} CH_3\overset{O}{\overset{\|}{C}}H \xrightarrow{CrO_3 \text{ or } KMnO_4} CH_3COOH$$

$CH_3COOH \xrightarrow{LiAlH_4} CH_3CH_2OH$

$CH_3CH_2OH \xrightarrow{KMnO_4} CH_3COOH$

(b) Reduction to Hydrocarbons (Wolff–Kishner Reduction)

$$\text{cyclohexanone} \xrightarrow[\text{Base}]{NH_2NH_2} \text{cyclohexane}$$

(c) Grignard Reactions

$$CH_3\overset{O}{\overset{\|}{C}}CH_3 + CH_3CH_2MgBr \xrightarrow{H_2O} CH_3\underset{CH_2CH_3}{\overset{OH}{C}}CH_3$$

(d) Cyanohydrin Formation

$$\text{cyclopentanone} \xrightarrow[H^+]{CN^-} \text{1-hydroxycyclopentane-1-carbonitrile (OH, CN)}$$

g. Carboxylic Acids

1. Preparation

(a) Oxidation of Primary Alcohols and Aldehydes

$$CH_3CH_2CH_2OH \xrightarrow{CrO_3} CH_3CH_2\overset{O}{\overset{\|}{C}}H \xrightarrow{CrO_3} CH_3CH_2COOH$$

$CH_3CH_2CH_2OH \xrightarrow{KMnO_4} CH_3CH_2COOH$

(b) Carbonation of Grignard Reagents

$$CH_3Br \xrightarrow[Et_2O]{Mg} CH_3MgBr \xrightarrow[H^+]{CO_2} CH_3COOH$$

HIGH-YIELD FACTS

(c) Hydrolysis of Nitriles

$$\text{C}_6\text{H}_{11}\text{Br} \xrightarrow{\text{NaCN}} \text{C}_6\text{H}_{11}\text{CN} \xrightarrow[\text{H}_2\text{O}]{\text{H}^+} \text{C}_6\text{H}_{11}\text{COOH}$$

2. Reactions

(a) Conversion to Functional Derivatives

$$CH_3CH_2COOH \xrightarrow[\text{or } PCl_3]{SOCl_2} CH_3CH_2\overset{O}{\overset{\|}{C}}Cl$$

$$CH_3CH_2COOH \xrightarrow[H^+]{C_6H_5OH} CH_3CH_2\overset{O}{\overset{\|}{C}}O{-}C_6H_5$$

$$CH_3CH_2COOH \xrightarrow[(2)NH_3]{(1)SOCl_2} CH_3CH_2\overset{O}{\overset{\|}{C}}NH_2$$

(b) Reduction

$$CH_3CH_2COOH \xrightarrow{NaBH_4} CH_3CH_2\overset{O}{\overset{\|}{C}}H \xrightarrow{NaBH_4} CH_3CH_2CH_2OH$$

$$CH_3CH_2COOH \xrightarrow{LiAlH_4} CH_3CH_2CH_2OH$$

h. Acyl Halides

1. Preparation

From Carboxylic Acids

$$CH_3CH_2COOH \xrightarrow{SOCl_2} CH_3CH_2\overset{O}{\overset{\|}{C}}Cl$$

2. Reactions

(a) Conversion to Carboxylic Acids and Carboxylic Acid Derivatives

$$CH_3CH_2\overset{O}{\overset{\|}{C}}Cl \xrightarrow{H_2O} CH_3CH_2COOH$$

$$CH_3CH_2\overset{O}{\overset{\|}{C}}Cl \xrightarrow{2NH_3} CH_3CH_2\overset{O}{\overset{\|}{C}}NH_2 + NH_4Cl$$

$$CH_3CH_2\overset{O}{\overset{\|}{C}}Cl \xrightarrow{CH_3OH} CH_3CH_2\overset{O}{\overset{\|}{C}}OCH_3$$

(b) Friedel–Crafts Acylation

$$CH_3CH_2\overset{O}{\overset{\|}{C}}Cl + C_6H_6 \xrightarrow{AlCl_3} C_6H_5\text{—}\overset{O}{\overset{\|}{C}}CH_2CH_3$$

(c) Reaction with Organolithium Compounds

$$CH_3Li \xrightarrow{CuBr} (CH_3)_2CuLi \xrightarrow{C_6H_5\text{—}\overset{O}{\overset{\|}{C}}\text{—}Cl} C_6H_5\text{—}\overset{O}{\overset{\|}{C}}\text{—}CH_3$$

i. Esters

1. Preparation

(a) From Alcohols and Carboxylic Acids

$$CH_3COOH + CH_3CH_2OH \underset{}{\overset{H^+}{\rightleftharpoons}} CH_3\overset{O}{\overset{\|}{C}}OCH_2CH_3$$

(b) From Acyl Halides

$$CH_3\overset{O}{\overset{\|}{C}}Cl + C_6H_5\text{—}OH \longrightarrow CH_3\overset{O}{\overset{\|}{C}}O\text{—}C_6H_5$$

2. Reactions

(a) Conversion to Carboxylic Acids (Hydrolysis), Amides (Ammonolysis), and Other Esters (Transesterification)

$$CH_3\overset{O}{\overset{\|}{C}}OCH_2CH_3 \xrightarrow[H^+]{H_2O} CH_3COOH + CH_3CH_2OH$$

$$CH_3\overset{O}{\overset{\|}{C}}OCH_2CH_3 \xrightarrow{NH_3} CH_3\overset{O}{\overset{\|}{C}}NH_2 + CH_3CH_2OH$$

$$CH_3\overset{O}{\overset{\|}{C}}OCH_2CH_3 \xrightarrow[H^+]{C_6H_5\text{—}OH} CH_3\overset{O}{\overset{\|}{C}}O\text{—}C_6H_5 + CH_3CH_2OH$$

(b) Reactions with Grignard Reagents

$$CH_3\overset{O}{\overset{\|}{C}}OCH_2CH_3 + 2\ CH_3\underset{MgBr}{\underset{|}{C}H}CH_3 \longrightarrow CH_3\overset{OH}{\overset{|}{\underset{CH(CH_3)_2}{\underset{|}{C}}}}\text{—}CH(CH_3)_2$$

(c) Reduction

$$CH_3\overset{O}{\overset{\|}{C}}OCH_2CH_3 \xrightarrow[\text{or } LiAlH_4,\ Et_2O,\ H_2O]{Ni,\ H_2} 2\ CH_3CH_2OH$$

$$CH_3\overset{O}{\overset{\|}{C}}OCH_3 \xrightarrow[\text{or } LiAlH_4,\ Et_2O,\ H_2O]{Ni,\ H_2} CH_3CH_2OH + CH_3OH$$

Cyclic lactone $\xrightarrow[\text{or } LiAlH_4,\ Et_2O,\ H_2O]{Ni,\ H_2}$ OH–$(CH_2)_5$–OH

j. Aromatic Compounds

Reactions

1. Electrophilic Aromatic Substitution

Benzene $\xrightarrow[H_2SO_4]{HONO_2}$ C_6H_5–NO_2 $\xrightarrow[\text{or Fe/HCl}]{H_2,\text{ catalyst}}$ C_6H_5–NH_2 $\xrightarrow{HONO}$ C_6H_5–N_2^+ Diazonium Salt

Benzene $\xrightarrow[H_2SO_4]{SO_3}$ C_6H_5–SO_3H $\xrightarrow[H_2O]{H^+}$ Benzene

Benzene $\xrightarrow[\text{Fe or } FeBr_3]{Br_2}$ C_6H_5–Br $\xrightarrow[Et_2O]{Mg}$ C_6H_5–MgBr $\xrightarrow[H_2O]{CO_2}$ C_6H_5–COOH

Benzene $\xrightarrow[AlCl_3]{CH_3CH_2Br}$ C_6H_5–CH_2CH_3

Benzene $\xrightarrow[AlCl_3]{CH_3\overset{O}{\overset{\|}{C}}Cl}$ C_6H_5–$\overset{O}{\overset{\|}{C}}CH_3$

2. Reactions Involving Diazonium Salts

Benzene $\xrightarrow[H_2SO_4]{HONO_2}$ C_6H_5–NO_2 $\xrightarrow[HCl]{Fe}$ C_6H_5–NH_2 $\xrightarrow{HONO}$ C_6H_5–N_2^+

C_6H_5–N_2^+ $\xrightarrow{H_3PO_2}$ Benzene

C_6H_5–N_2^+ $\xrightarrow{H^+}$ C_6H_5–OH

C_6H_5–N_2^+ $\xrightarrow{CuCl}$ C_6H_5–Cl

C_6H_5–N_2^+ $\xrightarrow{CuBr}$ C_6H_5–Br

C_6H_5–N_2^+ $\xrightarrow{CuCN}$ C_6H_5–CN $\xrightarrow{H_2O}$ C_6H_5–COOH

C_6H_5–N_2^+ $\xrightarrow{KI}$ C_6H_5–I

C_6H_5–N_2^+ $\xrightarrow[\text{Heat}]{HBF_4}$ C_6H_5–F

H Biology

1 DIFFERENCES BETWEEN PROKARYOTES AND EUKARYOTES

a. Characteristics of Prokaryotes

- Prokaryotes have no membrane-bound organelles (i.e., no nuclear membrane, no mitochondria, no lysosomes, no endoplasmic reticulum).
- Transcription and translation can occur at the same time (because no nuclear membrane or nucleus is present to separate the two processes).
- Ribosomes are 70S (composed of 30S and 50S ribosomal subunits).
- Prokaryotes have peptidoglycan cell walls, which is the site of action of many antibacterial drugs (e.g., penicillins, cephalosporins).
- Most adenosine triphosphate (ATP) synthesis occurs at the cell membrane (because prokaryotes lack mitochondria).
- Prokaryotes have no true nucleus or nucleoid region where DNA is located (i.e., no nuclear membrane).
- Mechanisms of gene transfer in prokaryotes are transduction, transformation, and conjugation.
- Antibiotic resistance is transferred by conjugation via plasmids.

The differences between prokaryotes and eukaryotes enable specially designed antibiotics to selectively kill prokaryotic cells (i.e., bacteria) by inhibiting prokaryotic cell membrane synthesis, protein synthesis, transcription, and DNA replication.

b. Characteristics of Eukaryotes

- Eukaryotes have membrane-bound organelles (i.e., nuclear membrane, mitochondria, lysosomes, and endoplasmic reticulum).
- Transcription and translation must occur independently (transcription takes place in the nucleus and translation takes place in the ribosomes).
- Ribosomes are 80S (composed of 40S and 60S ribosomal subunits), except mitochondrial ribosomes, which are 70S.
- Eukaryotes may or may not have a cellulose cell wall.
- Most ATP synthesis occurs in the mitochondria.

c. Table 2-11 shows a comparison of prokaryotes and eukaryotes.

2 VIRUSES

a. Definition

Viruses are obligate intracellular parasites; that is, they cannot live outside a host. A virus uses the metabolic machinery of its host to replicate. Viruses have no or-

TABLE 2-11. Comparison of prokaryotes and eukaryotes

Feature	Prokaryotes	Eukaryotes
Organelles	Absent	Present
Nucleus	Absent	Present
Nucleolus	Absent	Present
Genetic information	Single chromosomes[‡]	Multiple chromosomes
DNA	Naked	Packaged with proteins
Cell division	Cleavage/binary fission	Mitosis and meiosis
Protein synthesis	Coupled to transcription in the same compartment	RNA made in the nucleus; translated in the cytoplasm
Metabolism (primary)	Anaerobic and aerobic	Aerobic
Respiratory enzymes	Plasma membrane	Mitochondria
Cell wall	Present	Extracellular matrix
Cytoskeleton	Absent	Present
Endocytosis* or exocytosis[†]	Absent	Present

*Endocytosis is the process by which cells acquire extracellular materials by an invagination of the plasma membrane.
[†]Exocytosis is the process by which cells discard intracellular materials, and it occurs via fusion of intracellular vesicles with the plasma membrane.
[‡]A chromosome refers to a single molecule of DNA, and its associated proteins, that contains many genes.
Reprinted with permission from Davidson VL, Sittman DB: *NMS Biochemistry*, 3rd ed. Baltimore, Williams & Wilkins, 1994, p 92.

ganelles. Viruses that inhabit animals are called animal viruses, viruses that infect plants are called plant viruses, and viruses that infect bacteria are called bacteriophages (or phages for short).

Viruses consist of nucleic acid and enzymes encased in a protein coat.

Viruses consist of:

- Protein coat (both an inner and outer protein coat or only an inner coat)
- Nucleic acid (either DNA or RNA, but not both)
- Envelope (lipoprotein membrane that surrounds the protein coat) can be found on some viruses.

Retroviruses (e.g., HIV) can make DNA from RNA (reverse transcription) and contain the enzyme reverse transcriptase.

b. Life Cycle

1. **Sequences.** A virus can follow one of three sequences in its life cycle.
   (a) **Lytic cycle.** A virus undergoing a lytic cycle attaches to the plasma membrane of the cell it is infecting, releases its nucleic acid material into the cell, replicates, and transcribes its nucleic acid material. Some RNA viruses can transcribe mRNA from their RNA directly, whereas others (retroviruses) reverse-transcribe the RNA to DNA right after it enters the cell. In either case, the virus makes many copies of its genome (DNA or RNA) and translates many copies of the viral proteins necessary for the protein

coat(s). The cellular machinery is then used to assemble hundreds to thousands of viruses. Once a sufficient number of viruses have been constructed, the cell lyses and the viruses are released into the environment (i.e., the bloodstream) to infect other cells. This cycle always ends in cell death.

(b) **Lysogenic cycle.** In this cycle, the virus, after attaching to the plasma membrane and injecting its genetic material into the cell, integrates its genetic material into the host cell's genome or, alternatively, can persist in the cell as an extrachromosomal plasmid. The virus can thus lie dormant for many rounds of cell division, replicating its genetic material when the host cell replicates and never producing any new viruses or killing the host cell. In some instances, the virus can even give the host cell a survival advantage by passing on resistance to antibiotics or heavy metals (very useful in bacterial molecular biology).

Many viruses that enter the lysogenic cycle switch to the lytic cycle in a process known as **lytic induction;** this switch to an active phase is often in response to extracellular stress or DNA damage. In this situation, the virus makes new viruses and lyses the host cell as would any normal lytic virus.

(c) **Chronic infection.** In these cases (e.g., HIV or bacteriophage M13), the virus can enter a mixed stage called chronic or persistent infection. The virus does not kill the cell, but viruses are made and released at the plasma membrane surface through a budding process, the least common of the three types of viral life cycles.

2. **Switching Between Cycles.** A few viruses, such as bacteriophage lambda or hepatitis, can switch between the lytic and lysogenic (or even chronic infection) cycle (Figure 2-26); those viruses with more flexibility in their life cycle have a definite survival advantage. A virus that can choose between the lytic and lysogenic cycles can regulate the number of cells it kills per unit time, which allows the host organism to survive while a number of cells are lysed to release new viruses.

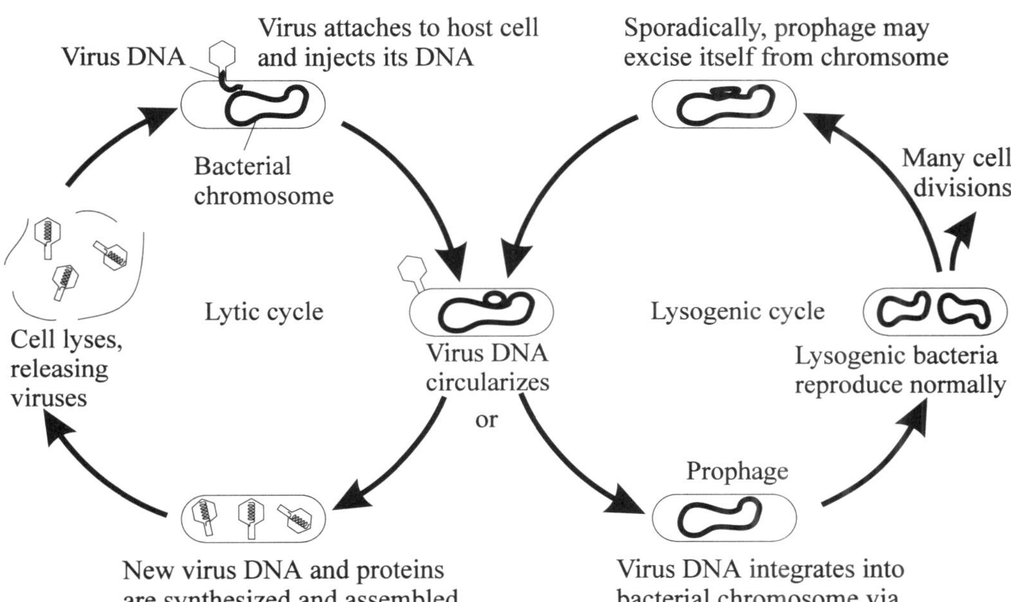

Figure 2-26.
The lytic and lysogenic cycles of bacteriophage lambda.

3 ORGANELLES AND MEMBRANE TRANSPORT (TABLE 2-12)

TABLE 2-12. Organelles and their functions

Organelle	Function
Ribosome	Is the site of protein synthesis (translation)
Rough endoplasmic reticulum (RER)	Has ribosomes bound to it, therefore functioning in the synthesis, chemical modification, and ultimate secretion of proteins
Smooth endoplasmic reticulum (SER)	Is the site of steroid synthesis and detoxification of drugs and poisons
Sarcoplasmic reticulum	Has voltage-dependent calcium channels used for muscle contraction. This specialized type of smooth endoplasmic reticulum is found in all types of muscle cells that sequester calcium ions.
Golgi apparatus	Receives proteins from the endoplasmic reticulum. Site of protein modification, packaging, and secretion
Lysosomes	Contain enzymes for the digestion of endocytosed particles and old organelles
Mitochondria	Is the site of the majority of ATP synthesis. (The Krebs cycle, electron transport chain, and oxidative phosphorylation all occur in the mitochondria.)
Centrioles	Participate in cell division (mitosis and meiosis)
Nucleus	Is the site of DNA replication and gene transcription
Nucleolus	Is the site of rRNA synthesis

a. Passive transport (simple diffusion)

[Figures 2-27 and 2-28; Table 2-13]. Molecules move down a gradient.

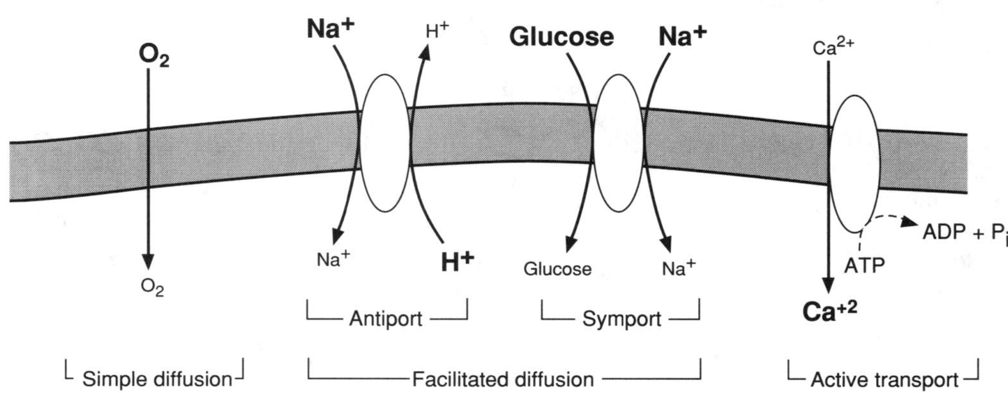

Figure 2-27. Membrane transport. In passive transport (simple diffusion), molecules move down a gradient. Facilitated, or carrier-mediated, transport exhibits saturation kinetics. Active transport moves a molecule up a concentration gradient, using ATP.

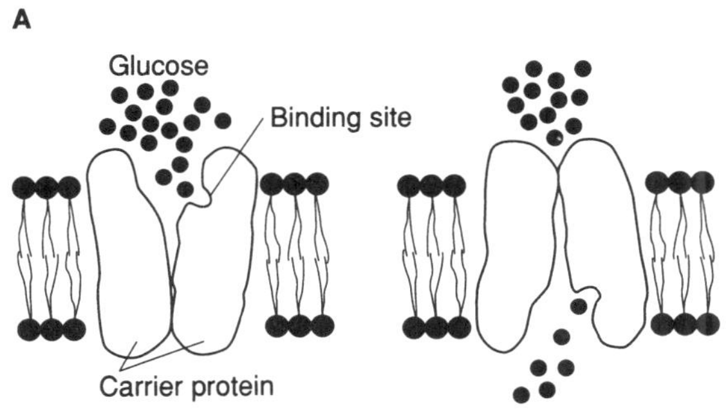

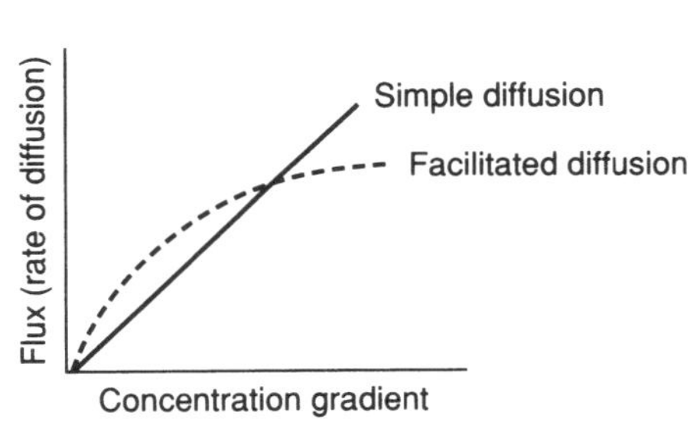

Figure 2-28. *(A)* The transmembrane carrier protein responsible for the facilitated diffusion of glucose undergoes a conformational change when glucose binds to it. The conformational change allows glucose to diffuse across the membrane down its concentration gradient. *(B)* In facilitated diffusion, the diffusion rate reaches a maximum when all the binding sites on the carrier protein are filled. Although the slope of the line may vary, the rate of membrane transport with simple diffusion is directly proportional to the concentration gradient of the molecule being transported, whereas facilitated (carrier-mediated) diffusion, like enzymes, exhibits saturation kinetics. (Reprinted with permission from Bullock J, Boyle J, Wang MB: *NMS Physiology,* 3rd ed. Baltimore, Williams & Wilkins, 1995, p 4.)

b. Facilitated, or carrier-mediated, transport.

Exhibits saturation kinetics (see Figure 2-28B).

c. Active transport

Molecules move up a concentration gradient, using ATP.

TABLE 2-13. Characteristics of different types of transport

Type	Electrochemical Gradient	Carrier-mediated	Metabolic Energy	Na^+ Gradient	Inhibition of Na^+-K^+ Pump
Simple diffusion	Downhill	No	No	No	
Facilitated diffusion	Downhill	Yes	No	No	
Primary active transport	Uphill	Yes	Yes		Inhibits (if Na^+-K^+ pump)
Cotransport	Uphill*	Yes	Indirect	Yes, same direction	Inhibits
Countertransport	Uphill*	Yes	Indirect	Yes, opposite direction	Inhibits

* One or more solutes are transported uphill; Na^+ is transported downhill.
Reprinted with permission from Bullock J, Boyle J, Wang MB: *NMS Physiology,* 3rd ed. Baltimore, Williams & Wilkins, 1995, p 4.

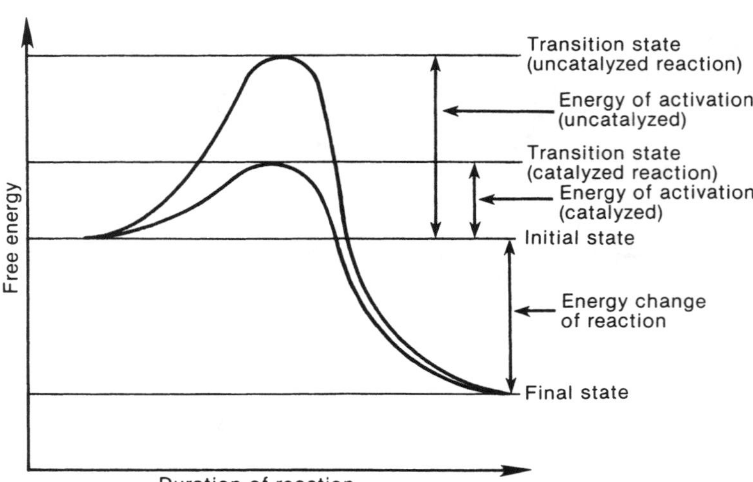

Figure 2-29. Diagrammatic representation of the free energy of activation of a chemical reaction. (Reprinted with permission from Davidson VL, Sittman DB: *NMS Biochemistry*, 3rd ed. Baltimore, Williams & Wilkins, 1994, p 87.)

4 ENZYME KINETICS AND CATALYSIS

a. Definitions

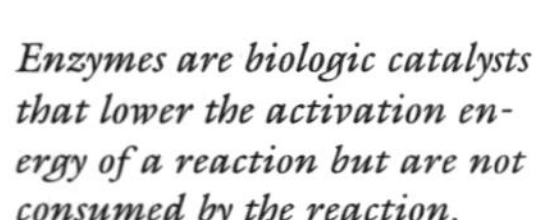
Enzymes are biologic catalysts that lower the activation energy of a reaction but are not consumed by the reaction.

Enzymes. Complex proteins that function as biologic catalysts, increasing the rate of both forward and reverse chemical reactions by lowering their energy of activation.

Enzymes do **not** change the free energy or the equilibrium constant of the reactions they catalyze (Figure 2-29)

Zymogen. An enzyme that is secreted in an inactive form that, under proper physiological conditions, undergoes proteolytic cleavage and is activated. Many digestive enzymes are secreted as zymogens to protect the intestinal organs from autodigestion (e.g., pepsinogen is secreted by chief cells of the stomach and is activated by H^+, which is secreted by the parietal cells of the stomach).

b. Enzyme Kinetics

$$E + S \underset{k_2}{\overset{k_1}{\rightleftharpoons}} ES \xrightarrow{k_{cat}} E + P$$

k_1 = rate of forward reaction
k_2 = rate of reverse reaction
k_{cat} = rate of catalyzed reaction
E = enzyme
S = substrate
ES = enzyme-substrate intermediate
P = product

c. Michaelis-Menten Equation

The Michaelis-Menten equation is used to describe the preceding reaction between an enzyme and a substrate. Do not memorize the derivation of this equation. Just understand why it produces the graph shown in Figure 2-30.

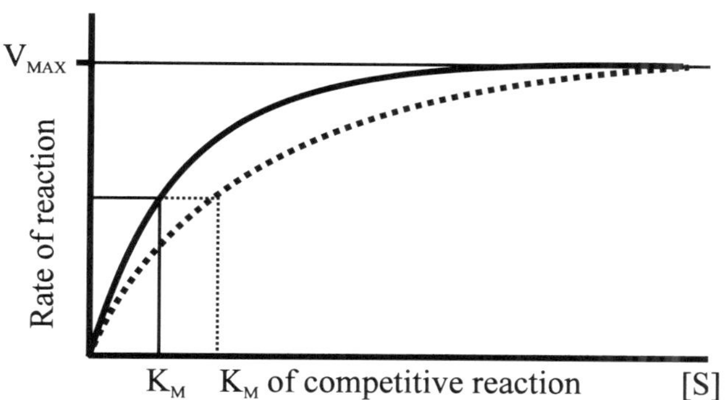

Figure 2-30. Enzyme kinetics. The *solid line* indicates an enzymatic reaction. The *dotted line* indicates an enzymatic reaction in the presence of a competitive inhibitor.

The final equation is as follows:

$$v = \frac{v_{max}[S]}{K_m + [S]}$$

v = reaction rate in forward direction

K_m = Michaelis-Menten constant for a given enzyme-catalyzed reaction

V_{max} = maximum rate of reaction (lots of substrate per molecule of enzyme)

[S] = concentration of substrate

The K_m is a very important concept; for when the concentration of substrate equals K_m, the reaction proceeds at half its maximal rate (which is a very efficient use of the enzyme). If the enzyme concentration is less than K_m, the enzyme is not used efficiently because there is too much substrate and not enough enzyme. On the other hand, if the enzyme concentration becomes larger than K_m, there will be too much free enzyme and not enough free substrate. For this reason, most enzymes in biologic systems tend to exist at concentrations close to K_m. An added benefit of having an enzyme concentration close to K_m is that small changes in the enzyme concentration have large effects on the speed of the reaction (since changes are on the steepest part of the curve), which makes it easier to regulate biologic reactions through the regulation of the enzyme concentration.

At low substrate concentrations, the rate of reaction depends primarily on the rate of formation of the enzyme–substrate complex (i.e., $k_{rxn} \approx k_1$).

Competitive inhibitors are substrates that inhibit an enzyme by binding to its active site. These substrates "compete" with the substrate inhibitors for the active site. Competitive inhibitors increase K_m but do not change the V_{max}. This type of inhibition can be overcome by increasing substrate concentration [S] (see Figure 2-30).

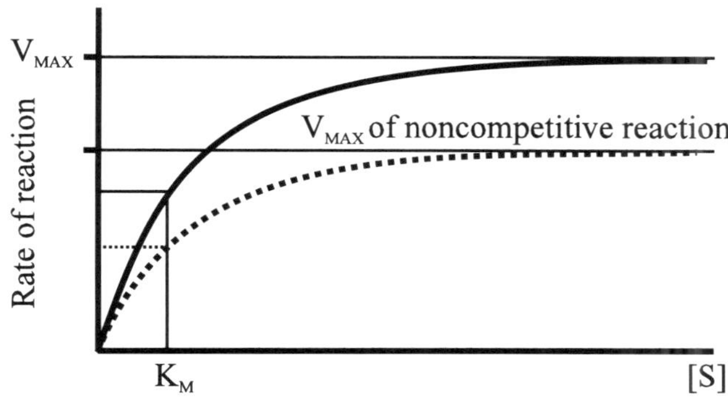

Figure 2-31. Effect of a noncompetitive inhibitor on enzyme kinetics. The *solid line* indicates an uninhibited enzymatic reaction. The *dotted line* indicates that an inhibitor accomplishes these effects by binding to the enzyme at a site other than its active site.

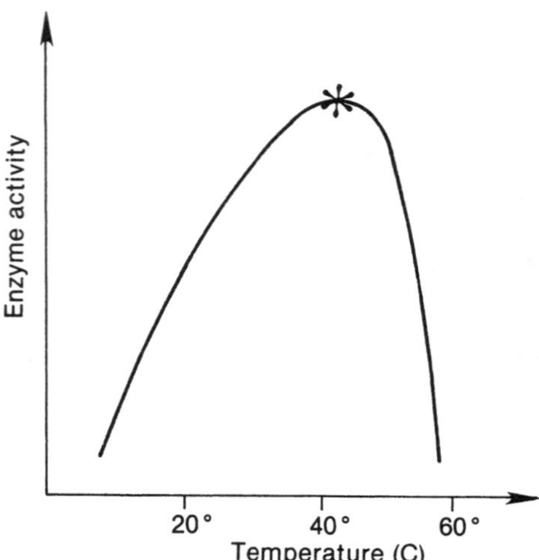

Figure 2-32.
Effect of temperature on the activity of an enzyme. The apparent optimum point shown here (*) is the result of an initial increase in reaction rate due to a rise in temperature, followed by a decrease in enzymatic activity as the temperature continues upward with increasing thermal denaturation of the proteinaceous enzyme molecule. (Reprinted with permission from Davidson VL, Sittman DB: *NMS Biochemistry,* 3rd ed. Baltimore, Williams & Wilkins, 1994, p 93.)

Noncompetitive inhibitors bind to a site other than the active site of the enzyme. This type of inhibitor does not prevent binding of the substrate to the active site of the enzyme. Noncompetitive inhibitors do not change K_m but decrease V_{max} (Figure 2-31).

Enzyme denaturation occurs at high temperatures, decreasing the rate of reaction at very high temperatures owing to thermal breakdown of the enzyme. Therefore, increasing the temperature increases the rate of an enzyme-catalyzed reaction to a certain extent, until the enzyme starts to denature, resulting in a decreased rate of reaction (Figures 2-32 and 2-33).

5 METABOLISM: BASIC PRINCIPLES

Organisms must use a series of reactions to metabolize (break down) organic molecules and release energy that can be used for biologic processes. The universal energy currency of the cell is **ATP.** Cells dephosphorylate ATP to adenosine diphosphate **(ADP)** and inorganic phosphate (P_i) in a reaction that releases approximately 7 kcal of energy per mole of ATP.

Although organisms can metabolize many different organic substrates to fulfill their energy requirements, sometimes the substrates are first converted to **glucose,** a

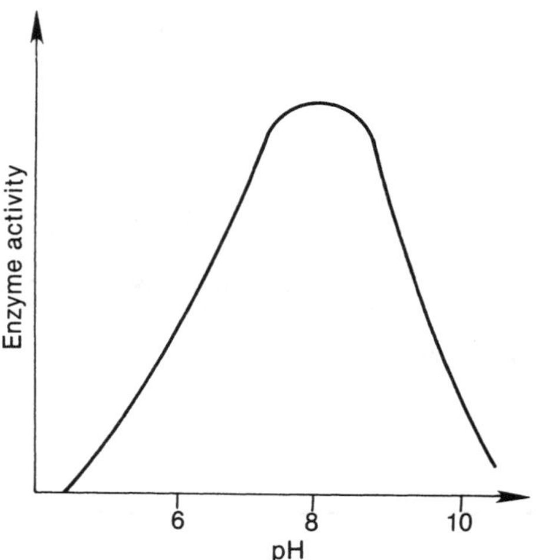

Figure 2-33.
A typical pH-activity plot of an enzyme-catalyzed reaction. (Reprinted with permission from Davidson VL, Sittman DB: *NMS Biochemistry,* 3rd ed. Baltimore, Williams & Wilkins, 1994, p 92.)

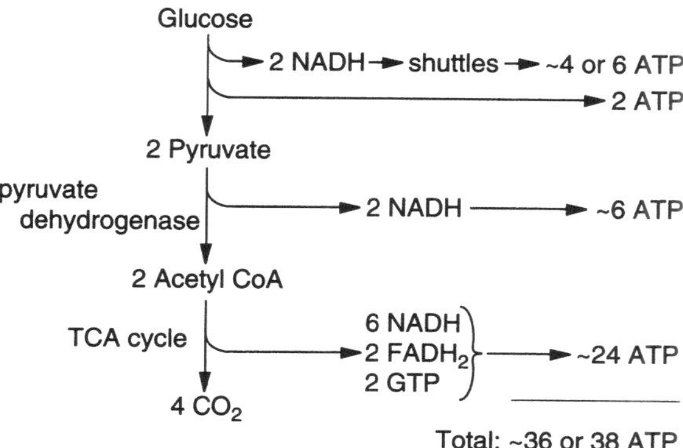

Figure 2-34. ATP produced by conversion of glucose to CO_2. The ATP produced by oxidative phosphorylation is approximate (indicated by ~). (Reprinted with permission from Marks DB: *BRS Biochemistry,* 2nd ed. Baltimore, Williams & Wilkins, 1994, p 156.)

hexose sugar that is the most common substrate catabolized by organisms. Consequently, you should focus your studies on the metabolism of glucose, although you should be aware that other reactions allow cells to metabolize substrates without conversion to glucose (such as the β-oxidation of fatty acids) [Figure 2-34].

The metabolism of glucose in eukaryotic (and many prokaryotic) cells is a complex series of reactions, described next. The MCAT frequently describes a part or all of the metabolism of glucose (possibly including a diagram); therefore, give yourself time to analyze the Krebs cycle so you can answer passage-based and discrete questions about the different steps.

TEST CORRELATION

a. Steps in Aerobic Respiration: Catabolism of Glucose

1. **Glycolysis**, which occurs in the cytosol, converts glucose to two molecules of pyruvic acid. See Figure 2-35 for the specific steps in this pathway. During glycolysis, two molecules of ATP are produced through substrate-level phosphorylation, a process that involves the direct coupling of a step in the catabolism of a substrate to the phosphorylation of an ADP molecule. In other words, the substrate is dephosphorylated and the ADP picks up the phosphate to form ATP. This process is not the most common method of ATP synthesis; most ATP is produced by oxidative phosphorylation via chemiosmotic coupling.

2. The **Krebs cycle** occurs in the mitochondrial matrix, which is the innermost part of the mitochondria (within the cristae). This cycle is also known as the citric acid or tricarboxylic acid (TCA) cycle (know all of these names). As the pyruvate molecules enter the mitochondrial matrix, they lose a carboxyl group and are converted to a two-carbon compound called acetyl coenzyme A, or acetyl CoA. Acetyl CoA then enters a circular series of reactions. In one turn of the Krebs cycle, two molecules of carbon dioxide are produced; they are in an oxidized state relative to acetyl CoA. One ATP is generated per turn, three molecules of NAD^+ are reduced to NADH, and one molecule of FAD is reduced to $FADH_2$ (for use in the electron transport chain). Note: One turn of the Krebs cycle is required for each acetyl CoA, so two turns of the

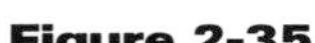

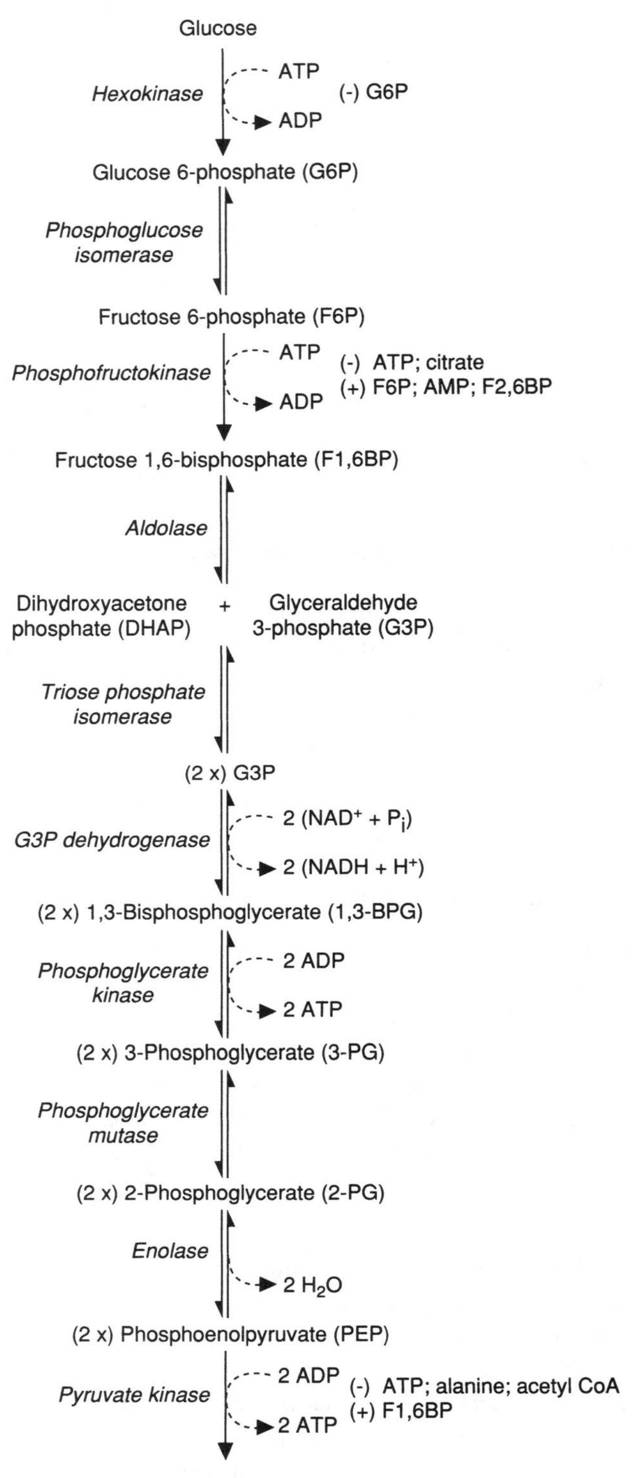

Figure 2-35.
The pathway of glycolysis. The signs (+) and (−) indicate the sites of action of allosteric positive and negative modulators of the activities of the key regulatory enzymes. (+) = activators; (−) = inhibitors; ADP = adenosine diphosphate; AMP = adenosine monophosphate; ATP = adenosine triphosphate; F2, 6BP = fructose 2,6-bisphosphate; NAD^+ = oxidized nicotinamide-adenine dinucleotide; NADH = reduced NAD; P_i = inorganic phosphate. (Reprinted with permission from Davidson VL, Sittman DB: *NMS Biochemistry*, 3rd ed. Baltimore, Williams & Wilkins, 1994, p 340.)

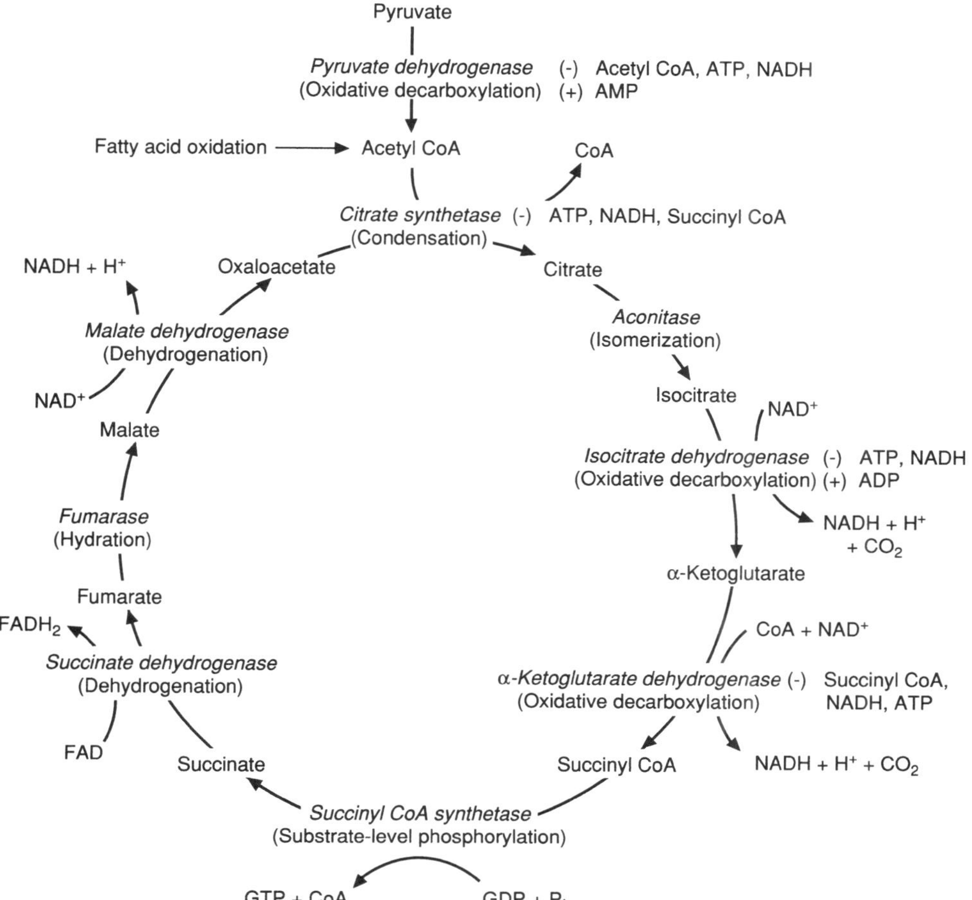

Figure 2-36. The reactions of pyruvate dehydrogenase and the Krebs cycle. The type of reaction that is catalyzed by each enzyme is indicated in *brackets* below the enzyme, which is indicated in *italic type*. Inhibitors and activators of regulatory enzymes are indicated by − and +, respectively. *ADP* = adenosine diphosphate; *AMP* = adenosine monophosphate; *ATP* = adenosine triphosphate; *CoA* = coenzyme A; *FAD* = flavin-adenine dinucleotide; *$FADH_2$* = reduced FAD; *GDP* = guanosine diphosphate; *GTP* = guanosine triphosphate; *NAD^+* = oxidized nicotinamide-adenine dinucleotide; *NADH* = reduced NAD; P_i = inorganic phosphate. (Reprinted with permission from Davidson VL, Sittman DB: *NMS Biochemistry,* 3rd ed. Baltimore, Williams & Wilkins, 1994, p 371.)

TCA cycle are required for each initial glucose molecule. See Figure 2-36 for details, but do not memorize it.

3. **Electron transport chain (ETC)/oxidative phosphorylation** occurs in the inner mitochondrial membrane. This stage of aerobic respiration requires oxygen. Most of the components of the electron transport chain are proteins that shift between oxidized and reduced states as they accept or release electrons. An important type of electron carrier is the **cytochrome**, which has a **heme** group that surrounds an iron atom. The electrons of NADH and $FADH_2$ are transferred to oxygen in an elegant series of reactions that produce energy and can in turn be used to phosphorylate ADP to ATP (Figure 2-37). For the MCAT, you need to know that before the ETC (as the electron transport chain is affectionately known), only four molecules of ATP have been produced (net production of 2 ATP because two are required for activation of reactants). During the ETC, another 34 molecules of ATP are produced (3 ATP per NADH, 2 ATP per $FADH_2$) with a cost of 2 ATP, for a net gain of 32 ATP in this step and 36 ATP overall.

b. Aerobic versus Anaerobic Respiration

The series of reactions previously discussed are entitled aerobic respiration because they require oxygen (the ETC) to metabolize glucose to completion. Some bacte-

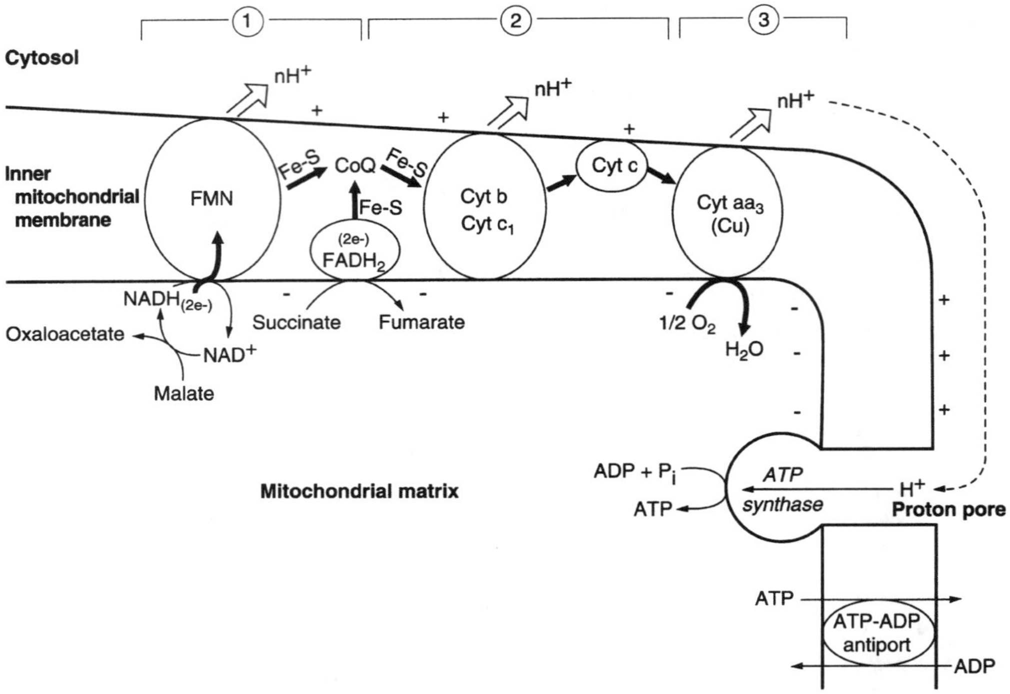

Figure 2-37. The electron transport chain and oxidative phosphorylation. *Heavy arrows* indicate the flow of electrons. *Fe-S* = iron-sulfur centers; FMN = flavin mononucleotide; CoQ = coenzyme Q (ubiquinone); Cyt = cytochrome. nH^+ indicates that an undetermined number of protons are pumped from the matrix to the cytosolic side. (Reprinted with permission from Marks DB: *BRS Biochemistry*, 2nd ed. Baltimore, Williams & Wilkins, 1994, p 118.)

ria cannot use oxygen, so what do they do? Or when eukaryotic cells run out of oxygen (e.g., muscle cells during strenuous exercise), what do they do?

Aerobic respiration yields 36 molecules of ATP, whereas anaerobic respiration yields only 2 molecules of ATP.

The answer is **anaerobic respiration** (the metabolism of glucose in the absence of oxygen). Whereas aerobic respiration consists of glycolysis, the Krebs cycle, and ETC/oxidative phosphorylation, anaerobic glycolysis involves glycolysis, then the conversion of pyruvate to lactic acid (or ethanol). Whereas aerobic respiration gives a net gain of 36 ATP, anaerobic respiration gives the cell only 2 ATP (no wonder eukaryotic cells choose aerobic respiration in the presence of oxygen). Unfortunately, not all bacteria have this luxury and have to subsist on anaerobic respiration, or fermentation, with an end product of either alcohol or lactic acid.

During strenuous exercise, muscle cells can run out of oxygen. Faced with no better option, these cells begin to anaerobically respire glucose to lactic acid, resulting in the buildup of an "oxygen debt." You can feel the "debt" when your muscles cramp and begin to burn as you work them hard. Once the muscles relax and again receive sufficient oxygen from the blood, the cells can "repay the oxygen debt" and convert the lactate back to pyruvate and continue with aerobic respiration.

6 ENZYME/HORMONE REGULATION

a. Definitions

1. **Covalent modification** usually involves the phosphorylation or dephosphorylation of specific enzymes and results in the activation or inactivation of that particular enzyme. For example, when insulin binds to its receptor, it triggers a series of events that lead first to the dephosphorylation of glycogen synthase

and, as a result, to its activation, thereby promoting glycogen synthesis and decreasing blood glucose levels.

2. **Allosteric effects** constitute the major method of enzymatic regulation and usually proceed by an enzymatic reaction in which the product binds to the enzyme at a site other than its active site to inhibit further activity of the enzyme (this reaction is known as feedback inhibition). The allosteric enzyme oscillates between an active conformation (the enzyme is capable of catalyzing the reaction) and an inactive conformation (the enzyme is incapable of catalyzing the reaction).

   Characteristics of allosteric modification (Figure 2-38)

   - It always involves an allosteric enzyme.
   - It is very rapid (unlike transcriptional regulation of enzymes).
   - It can result in enzymatic inhibition or activation.
   - It provides an efficient method of conserving cellular energy and avoids the accumulation of metabolic intermediates.

3. **Negative feedback** inhibition occurs when the end product of a pathway inhibits (i.e., negatively feeds back) an earlier enzyme/hormone on the pathway (Figure 2-39). It is the most common mechanism of hormone regulation.

Most hormones are regulated by negative feedback.

Figure 2-39 shows a classic example of a system with negative feedback. The secretion of corticotropin-releasing hormone (CRH) by the hypothalamus stimulates the secretion of ACTH by the anterior pituitary; then ACTH stimulates the secretion of cortisol into the bloodstream by the adrenal cortex. If too much cortisol is present, it inhibits further CRH secretion by the hypothalamus. Cortisol can inhibit ACTH secretion by the anterior pituitary if sufficient cortisol has already been secreted by the adrenal cortex in response to ACTH.

4. **Positive feedback** occurs when an end product stimulates the secretion or production of an earlier enzyme or hormone, which can lead to a continuous feedback cycle that escalates the levels of both chemicals. Positive feedback occurs during the menstrual cycle, when LH stimulates estrogen, which acts to further stimulate the secretion of LH, resulting in an **LH surge,** which triggers ovulation.

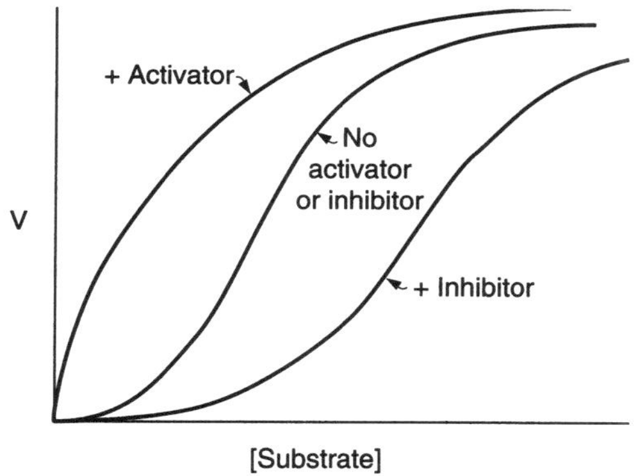

Figure 2-38. Effect of activators and inhibitors on an allosteric enzyme. (Reprinted with permission from Marks DB: *BRS Biochemistry,* 2nd ed. Baltimore, Williams & Wilkins, 1994, p 36.)

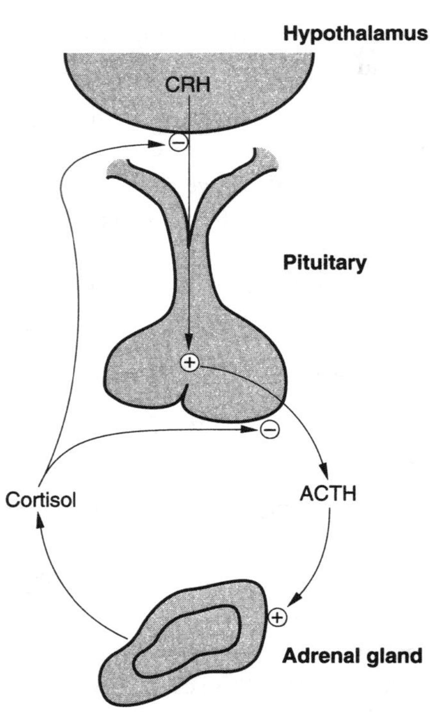

Figure 2-39. Hormone feedback regulation. *CRH* = corticotropin-releasing hormone; *ACTH* = adrenocorticotropic hormone; ⊕ = activates; ⊖ = inhibits. (Reprinted with permission from Marks DB: *BRS Biochemistry,* 2nd ed. Baltimore, Williams & Wilkins, 1994, p 285.)

b. Transcriptional Regulation of Enzymes

1. **Prokaryotic gene regulation** is largely at the level of transcription. The two most common instances of prokaryotic gene regulation follow.

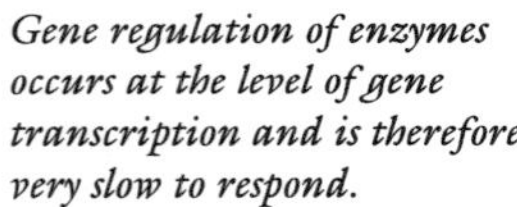
Gene regulation of enzymes occurs at the level of gene transcription and is therefore very slow to respond.

(a) **Operons** are found in bacteria but have not been found in eukaryotes. The most common example of an operon is the *lac* operon, which codes for enzymes that regulate the transport and metabolism of lactose (Figure 2-40). The *lac* **repressor** is a protein that is continuously made by the *lac* operon. In the absence of lactose, the *lac* repressor can tightly bind to the **operator** sequence of the *lac* operon. If the repressor is bound to the operator, RNA polymerase cannot bind to the **promoter** sequence and initiate transcription. On the other hand, if lactose is present in the cell, a molecule of lactose can bind to the repressor and prevent the repressor from binding to the operator sequence. RNA polymerase can now bind to the repressor protein and can therefore transcribe the *lac* operon genes (which code for the transport and metabolization of lactose) in an example of **negative transcriptional regulation.** One can easily imagine the opposite process, called **positive transcriptional regulation,** where the inducible substance (e.g., cAMP) can enhance RNA polymerase's ability to bind to the promoter sequence and initiate transcription.

(b) **Attenuation** is a much more complex process that uses the prokaryotic coupling of transcription and translation to regulate gene expression. The ribosome follows RNA polymerase closely; if it follows too closely, it will inhibit further transcription through the formation of a stem–loop complex. On the other hand, if it stalls because of lack of appropriate

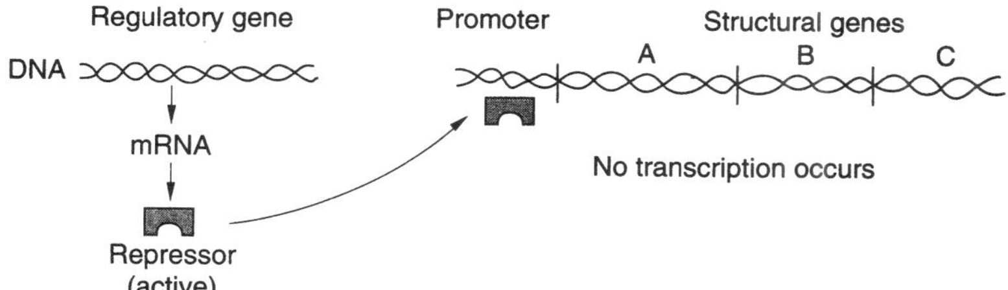

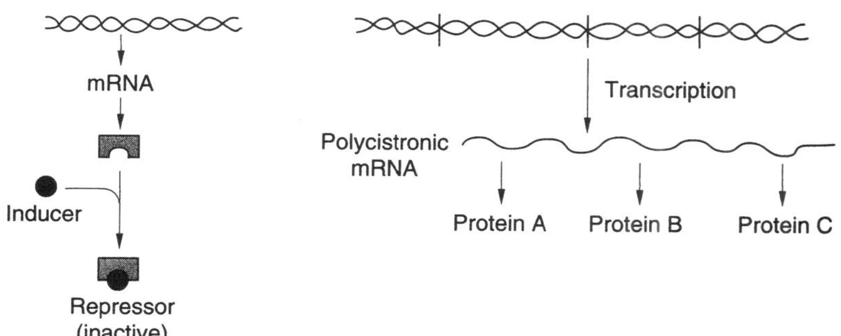

Figure 2-40.
An inducible operon (e.g., the *lac* operon). (Reprinted with permission from Marks DB: *BRS Biochemistry,* 2nd ed. Baltimore, Williams & Wilkins, 1994, p 75.)

amino acid tRNA complexes to attach to the codons, the RNA polymerase can continue transcribing and the gene is turned on. This process is used to regulate the gene transcription necessary for the synthesis of amino acids; these genes are turned on only when amino acid levels are low and the ribosome stalls. The most common example of attenuation is the **tryptophan (trp) operon.**

2. **Eukaryotic gene regulation** is much more complex and less well understood. Proteins called **transcription factors** can enhance transcription by binding to any of the following types of sequences:

   (a) **Promoters** are the sequence where the RNA polymerase binds. Many different transcription factors help RNA polymerase bind to the promoter, most notably TFIID (which binds to the upstream TATA box).

   (b) **Proximal promoter elements** are additional sequences that are located upstream of the transcriptional start site and enhance transcription within 200 nucleotides of the promoter.

   (c) **Enhancers** are sequences located far away from the transcriptional start site (greater than 200 nucleotides away, or even within or behind the gene) that increase transcriptional rates.

   (d) **Steroid hormones** can regulate gene transcription of enzymes by binding to steroid receptor elements (SREs) on DNA, which affect transcriptional activity.

   (e) **Chromatin structure** also affects gene transcription; genes within nucleosomes are not as likely to be transcribed as genes between nucleosomes.

In the disease congenital adrenal hyperplasia (CAH), the adrenal cortex is unable to make the hormone cortisol. Would the levels of ACTH be elevated or decreased in a patient with CAH?

ACTH levels would be **increased** in a patient with CAH owing to a lack of negative feedback caused by the absence of cortisol production.

7 MENDELIAN GENETICS

a. Locus

is a "gene"; the smallest unit of hereditary information.

b. Allele

is one genetic variant at a particular locus (e.g., A or a).

c. Genotype

is the genetic constitution of an individual at a particular locus (e.g., Aa).

d. Phenotype

is the physical appearance of an individual (e.g., bald, tall).

e. Homozygote

is an individual who has two identical alleles at the same locus (e.g., AA or aa).

f. Heterozygote

is an individual who has two different alleles at the same locus in different chromosomes (e.g., Aa).

g. Dominant

is the allele whose phenotype is expressed in the heterozygote.

h. Recessive

is the allele whose phenotype is not expressed in the heterozygote.

The classic phenotypic ratio of a monohybrid cross (Aa × Aa) = 3:1 (dominant:recessive), as shown in Figure 2-41. The classic phenotypic ratio of a dihybrid cross (AaBb × AaBb) is 9:3:3:1 (dominant/dominant; dominant/recessive; recessive/dominant; recessive/recessive) [see Figure 2-41].

A

	A	a
A	AA	Aa
a	Aa	aa

B

	AB	Ab	aB	ab
AB	AABB	AABb	AaBB	AaBb
Ab	AABb	AAbb	AaBb	Aabb
aB	AaBB	AaBb	aaBB	aaBb
ab	AaBb	Aabb	aaBb	aabb

Figure 2-41. *(A)* Monohybrid cross; *(B)* dihybrid cross.

i. A Pedigree

is a flowchart depicting the transmission or inheritance of a particular trait or disease through a particular family. Males are written as squares, females as circles. Dead people are sometimes written with slashes through the circle or square, with the age inserted below. When examining a pedigree, keep in mind the following rules:

1. First, look at the number of males versus the number of females affected. If almost all of the people who are affected are males, the disorder is **X-linked recessive** (X-linked dominant disorders are very rare). If every single one of the people who have the disorder is male, it could be Y-linked (e.g., hairy ear rims). Y-linked conditions are extremely rare and probably will not be mentioned on the MCAT.
2. Then, look at the parents. **If two normal parents have an affected child, the disorder is most likely autosomal recessive.** If an affected parent married to a nonaffected parent has 50% or more children who receive the trait in question, the disease is probably autosomal dominant.

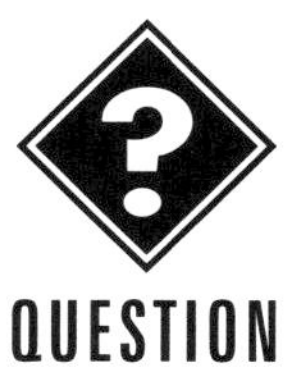

A man with a family history of red–green color blindness has the following pedigree:

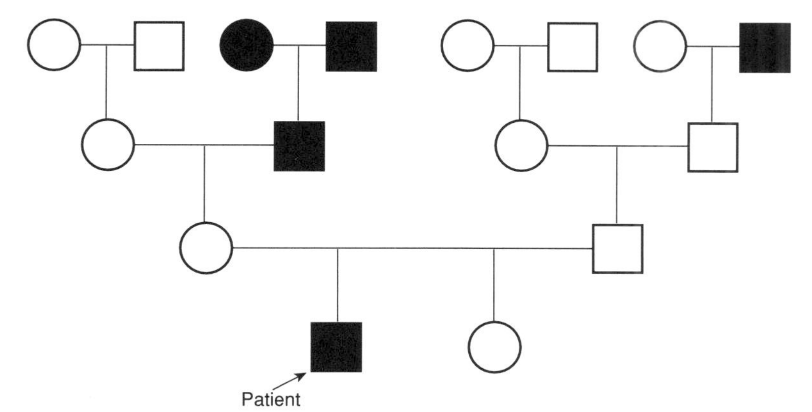

(a) What is the most likely mode of inheritance of red–green color blindness that reflects this patient's pedigree?
(b) What is the probability that the patient's sister is a carrier of the red–green color blindness trait?
(c) If the patient's sister marries a man who does *not* have red–green color blindness, what is the probability that their child will be color-blind?

ANSWER

(a) Because four males are affected and only one female is affected, and because two normal parents can have an affected child, the trait is most likely X-linked recessive.
(b) Using Punnett squares (X^a = color-blindness gene)

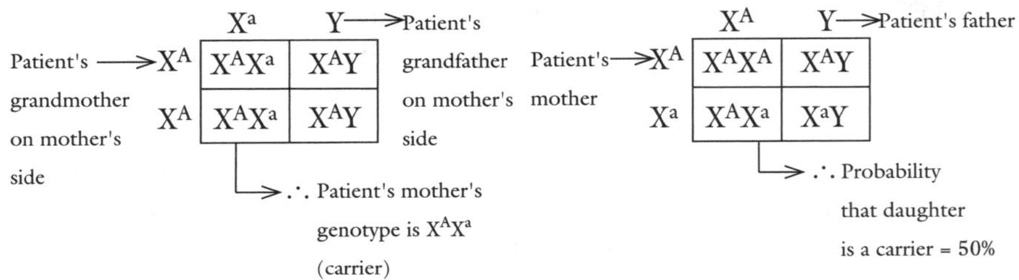

(c) The probability that their child will be color-blind

=P (daughter is a carrier) × P ($X^AX^a \times X^AY$ results in a color-blind child)

50% [see (b)] ×

	X^A	Y
X^A	X^AX^A	X^AY
X^a	X^AX^a	X^aY → color-blind

25%

Therefore, the probability that their child will be color-blind

$$= 50\% \times 25\% = 12.5\% = 1/8$$

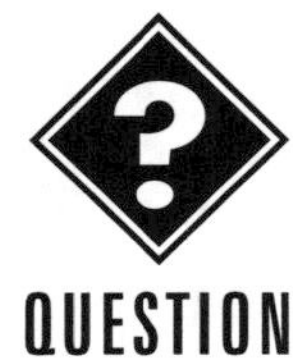

QUESTION

If a person with blood group O marries a person with blood group AB, what is the probability that their baby will have blood group O?

ABO blood grouping is an example of a **codominant trait:** blood groups A and B are both dominant, and blood group O is recessive.

Genotype	Phenotype
I^Ai or I^AI^A	A
I^Bi or I^BI^B	B
I^AI^B	AB
ii	O

Therefore, when the Punnett square for this problem is:

	I^A	I^B
i	I^Ai	I^Bi
i	I^Ai	I^Bi

the probability that their baby will be blood group O is 0%.

8 POPULATION GENETICS: HARDY-WEINBERG EQUILIBRIUM

a. Hardy-Weinberg Equilibrium

describes the genotype frequencies (called PIC values) and phenotype frequencies of a large population that has reached an equilibrium state.

$$p + q = 1$$

p = frequency of the dominant allele
q = frequency of the recessive allele

Squaring this equation results in the **Hardy-Weinberg equation:**

$$(p + q)^2 = p^2 + 2pq + q^2 = 1$$

p^2 = frequency of dominant homozygotes
2pq = frequency of heterozygotes
q^2 = frequency of recessive homozygotes

p = frequency of the dominant allele
q = frequency of the recessive allele

b. Assumptions of Hardy-Weinberg Equilibrium

- **Large population** is necessary to minimize the effects of "genetic drift" (the chance elimination of one allele owing to the small size of a population).
- **Random mating** is assumed: No natural selection or preferential mating to ensure that organisms with the preferred genotype are more likely to leave greater numbers of offspring.

HIGH-YIELD FACTS

- **No immigration or emigration** is assumed: Within the population, even a small amount of gene flow can affect a Hardy-Weinberg equilibrium.
- **No spontaneous mutations.**

QUESTION

Cystic fibrosis is an autosomal recessive disease that affects 16% of the people in a given population. Assuming that the population is in Hardy-Weinberg equilibrium, what percentage of heterozygous carriers has the cystic fibrosis gene?

ANSWER

$$q^2 = 0.16$$

$$q = 0.4$$

Since

$$p + q = 1$$

$$p = 0.6$$

Using the Hardy-Weinberg equation:

$$p^2 + 2pq + q^2 = 1$$

where $2pq$ = number of heterozygous carriers, the answer is 2(0.6)(0.4) = 48%

9 MOLECULAR BIOLOGY OF DNA AND RNA

a. DNA (Deoxyribonucleic Acid)

A = T has 2 H-bonds

G ≡ C has 3 H-bonds

Adenine and guanine are double-ringed purines, whereas cytosine, uracil, and thymine are single-ringed pyrimidines.

In 1953, Watson and Crick worked out the structure of DNA and RNA using x-ray crystallography. DNA is composed of a 2′-deoxyribose and base pairs A–T, C–G (A = adenine, T = thymine, C = cytosine, G = guanine, and U = uracil; uracil is found only in RNA, and thymine is found only in DNA). It is arranged into a double helix, with the nucleic acid–base pairs in the center, which are connected to the sugar–phosphate backbone (Figure 2-42). The three types of DNA are A, B, and Z; most DNA in eukaryotic nuclei is in the B–DNA conformation. B–DNA has approximately 10 base pairs per turn of the double helix, and the helix has major and minor grooves (in B–DNA). The major grooves are bigger than the minor grooves.

The DNA replication process is catalyzed by the enzyme DNA polymerase. The process has been duplicated in vivo and is well understood. **DNA replication is semiconservative,** as this was demonstrated by the Meselson-Stahl labeling experiment. The parent DNA breaks into two separate single strands, which can then

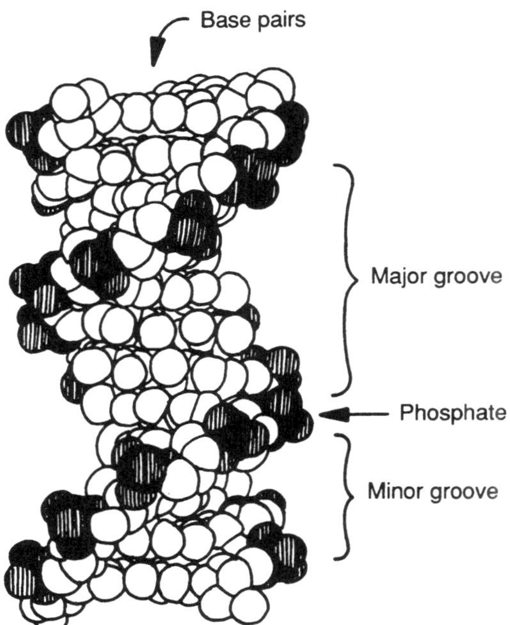

Figure 2-42.
The DNA double helix. (Reprinted with permission from Marks DB: *BRS Biochemistry,* 2nd ed. Baltimore, Williams & Wilkins, 1994, p 52.)

serve as templates for DNA polymerase to add nucleotides and make two new daughter strands (each of which has half of the parent strand). DNA synthesis occurs in the 5′ → 3′ direction (these directions are defined by the directionality of the deoxyribose–phosphate bond). One daughter strand is replicated continuously, but the other daughter strand must be synthesized in a series of **Okazaki segments.** In addition to DNA polymerase, a number of enzymes contribute to DNA replication, including DNA ligase, which connects Okazaki segments. DNA replication begins at specific sites with the formation of **replication forks.**

The leading strand of DNA is synthesized in a continuous fashion, whereas the lagging strand is synthesized in a discontinuous fashion involving the synthesis and ligation of multiple Okazaki fragments.

b. RNA (Ribonucleic Acid)

RNA is composed of a ribose sugar, phosphate, and base pairs **A-U** (instead of A-T), C-G. Unlike DNA, **RNA is single-stranded** and very unstable. The three major types of RNA are:

1. **rRNA**—ribosomal RNA. This type of RNA makes up ribosomes and is the most abundant form of RNA in vivo.
2. **mRNA**—messenger RNA. This type is transcribed from DNA in the nucleus and translated into proteins in ribosomes in the cytoplasm. Heterogeneous nuclear RNA (hnRNA) is a predecessor that is modified to form mRNA by intron splicing. mRNA is the largest type of RNA in vivo.
3. **tRNA**—transfer RNA (Figure 2-43). tRNA are small RNA molecules that can match specific amino acids to specific mRNA triplet nucleotide sequences (codons). Specificity is the basis for the genetic code. It is important to remember that there are three termination (stop) codons (UAA, UAG, UGA), one initiation codon (AUG = methionine), and 60 other codons. Therefore, **more than one codon can be present for a particular amino acid;** most of the degeneracy in the genetic code is in the third nucleotide of the codon. tRNA is the smallest type of RNA in vivo.

Figure 2-43.
The cloverleaf structure of tRNA. Bases that commonly occur in a particular position are indicated by *letters*. Base-pairing in stem regions is indicated by *lines* between strands. Ψ = pseudouridine; *T* = ribothymidine; *D* = dihydrouridine. (Reprinted with permission from Marks DB: *BRS Biochemistry,* 2nd ed. Baltimore, Williams & Wilkins, 1994, p 55.)

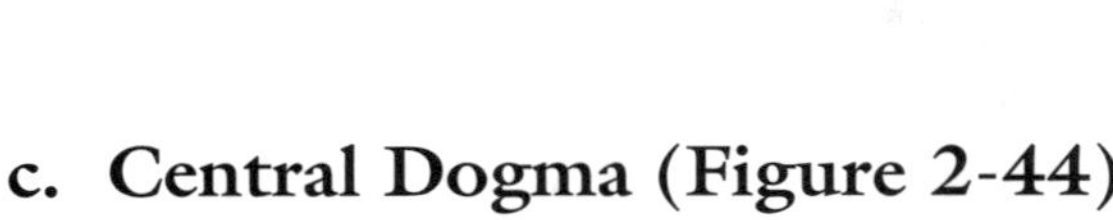

c. Central Dogma (Figure 2-44)

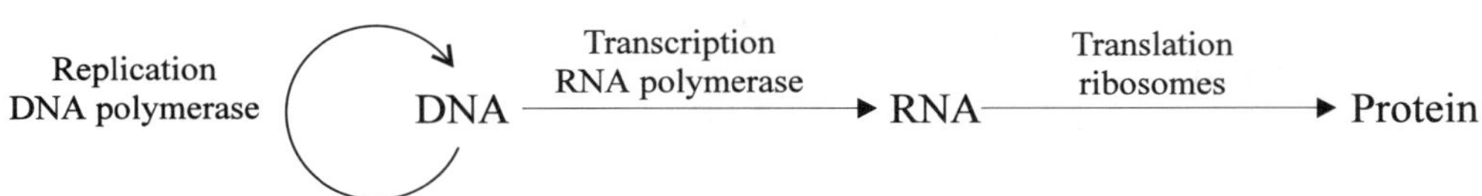

Figure 2-44.
The central premise of molecular biology.

Eukaryotic transcription occurs in the nucleus, whereas translation occurs in the cytosol on ribosomes.

All genetic information is stored as DNA (mostly in the nucleus; mitochondria and chloroplasts have their own DNA). The "central premise" elucidates the process of genetic information transfer in all known organisms, from little *Escherichia coli* to the biggest eukaryotic organisms. DNA must first be transcribed to mRNA by RNA polymerase (specifically by RNA polymerase II) within the nucleus. The mRNA then leaves the nucleus (in eukaryotes) and travels to the ribosomes, where it is translated to protein. The ribosome subunits recruit the proper tRNAs, which can bond to the mRNA codons and carry the proper amino acids. The amino acids are joined via peptide bonds to create a protein. As a result, all genetic information is transmitted through the formation of proteins, which catalyze reactions, form structural macromolecules, and initiate all other important cellular functions.

The central premise has two important exceptions.

- One occurs in **retroviruses,** which carry their information as RNA, which can then reverse-transcribe to DNA via the enzyme **reverse transcriptase** (the DNA is then transcribed as normal). Molecular biologists have used reverse transcriptase to make cDNA from eukaryotic mRNA, which has the genes without the promoters, introns, and so forth (which makes them easier to manipulate in bacterial systems).
- Other RNA viruses can use RNA-dependent RNA polymerases to turn their RNA information directly into translatable mRNA.

In eukaryotes, transcription occurs in the nucleus and translation occurs in the cytoplasm on ribosomes. Because prokaryotes do not have a nuclear membrane, the processes of transcription and translation are coupled and occur simultaneously.

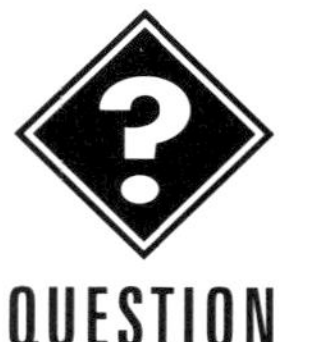

Look at the following nucleotide:

(a) Is this nucleotide found in DNA or RNA?

(b) This nucleotide contains all of the following organic functional groups EXCEPT:

 (1) Alkene
 (2) Alcohol
 (3) Ether
 (4) Ester
 (5) Amide

(c) If the content of adenine in a piece of double-stranded DNA is 30% of the total nitrogenous bases, what is the percentage of guanine?

(a) Because an -OH group is present on the 2′ position of the ribose sugar (see below), this nucleotide is only present in RNA.

(b) The answer is **4.** The functional groups are outlined in the figure below:

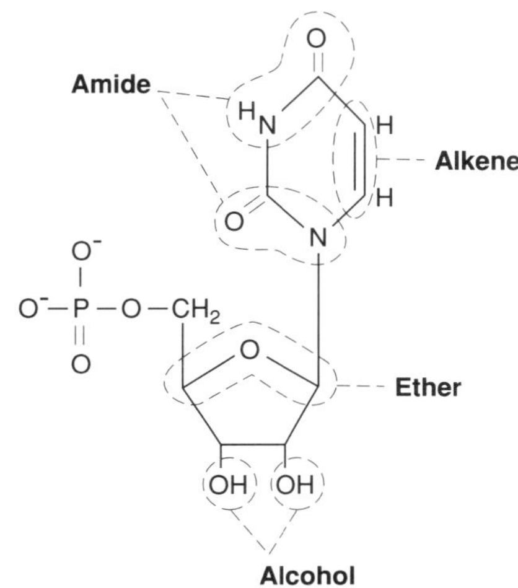

(c) In a piece of double-stranded DNA, adenine base pairs with thymine and cytosine base pairs with guanine. The percentage of adenine (i.e., 30%) is equal to the percentage of thymine. If the percentage of adenine plus thymine equals 60%, then the percentage of guanine plus cytosine equals 40%. The percentage of guanine (i.e., 20%) is equal to the percentage of cytosine.

10 AMINO ACIDS AND PROTEIN STRUCTURE

Table 2-14 lists amino acids and the group to which each belongs. Structures of the amino acids are shown in Figure 2-45.

a. Amino Acids: Distinguishing Characteristics

- Arginine is the most alkaline (basic) amino acid.
- Glycine is the only achiral amino acid. All other amino acids are optically active.

Positively charged amino acids (lysine, histidine) can be found on histone proteins, allowing the histones to interact with DNA. DNA carries an enormous negative charge because of its phosphate backbone.

TABLE 2-14. Amino acid groups

Group	Amino Acids
Acidic [Negatively charged: R-COO$^-$]	Aspartate (Asp) Glutamate (Glu)
Basic [Positively charged: R-NH$_3^+$]	Arginine (Arg) Lysine (Lys) Histidine (His)
Alipathic side chain	Glycine (Gly) Alanine (Ala) *Valine (Val) *Leucine (Leu) *Isoleucine (Ile)
Aromatic side chain	Tyrosine (Tyr) *Phenylalanine (Phe) Tryptophan (Trp)
Amide-containing	Asparagine (Asn) Glutamine (Gln)
Sulfur-containing	Cysteine (Cys) *Methionine (Met)
-OH-containing alipathic	Serine (Ser) Threonine (Thr)
Cyclic imino acid (C=N link)	Proline (Pro)

*These hydrophobic amino acids are typically found on the inside of the protein (away from the periphery, which is usually in contact with water).

A

$^{-}OOC-C(H)(NH_3^+)-R = \vdash R$

	R		R
Glycine (Gly; G)	$\vdash H$	**Serine** (Ser; S)	$\vdash CH_2-OH$
Alanine (Ala; A)	$\vdash CH_3$	**Threonine** (Thr; T)	$\vdash CH(OH)-CH_3$
Valine (Val; V)	$\vdash CH(CH_3)-CH_3$	**Phenylalanine** (Phe; F)	$\vdash CH_2-C_6H_5$
Leucine (Leu; L)	$\vdash CH_2-CH(CH_3)-CH_3$	**Tryptophan** (Trp; W)	$\vdash CH_2-$(indole, N–H)
Isoleucine (Ile; I)	$\vdash CH(CH_3)-CH_2-CH_3$	**Methionine** (Met; M)	$\vdash CH_2-CH_2-S-CH_3$
Asparagine (Asn; N)	$\vdash CH_2-C(=O)-NH_2$	**Glutamine** (Gin; Q)	$\vdash CH_2-CH_2-C(=O)-NH_2$

Proline (Pro; P) — CH_2-CH_2, CH_2, $CH-COO^-$, N^+H_2 (ring)

B

$HOOC-C(H)(NH_3^+)-R \xleftrightarrow{pk\approx3\ (\alpha\text{-carboxyl})} {}^{-}OOC-C(H)(NH_2)-R$; $pk\approx9$ (α-amino)

Amino acid	Below pK	pK	Above pK
Aspartic Acid (Asp; D)	$\vdash CH_2-C(=O)OH$	pK≈4	$\vdash CH_2-C(=O)O^- + H^+$
Glutamic Acid (Glu; E)	$\vdash CH_2-CH_2-C(=O)OH$	pK≈4	$\vdash CH_2-CH_2-C(=O)O^- + H^+$
Histidine (His; H)	$\vdash CH_2-C=C-NH-CH=N^+H$ (imidazolium) $+H^+$	pK≈6.5	$\vdash CH_2-C=C-NH-CH=N$ (imidazole) $+H^+$
Cysteine (Cys; C)	$\vdash CH_2-SH$	pK≈8	$\vdash CH_2-S^- + H^+$
Lysine (Lys; K)	$\vdash CH_2-CH_2-CH_2-CH_2-NH_3^+$	pK≈10	$\vdash CH_2-CH_2-CH_2-CH_2-NH_2 + H^+$
Tyrosine (Tyr; Y)	$\vdash CH_2-C_6H_4-OH$	pK≈10	$\vdash CH_2-C_6H_4-O^- + H^+$
Arginine (Arg; R)	$\vdash CH_2-CH_2-CH_2-NH-C(=NH_2^+)-NH_2$	pK≈12	$\vdash CH_2-CH_2-CH_2-NH-C(=NH)-NH_2 + H^+$

Figure 2-45.
Structures of the amino acids. Abbreviations are given for all amino acids. *(A)* shows amino acids that do not have ionizable side chains. *(B)* shows side chains that are ionizable. In *(B)*, for each amino acid, the species that predominates at a pH below the pK is shown on the *left;* the species that predominates at a pH above the pK is shown on the *right*. Note that the charge changes from 0 to − or from + to 0. At the pK, equal amounts of both species are present. (Reprinted with permission from Marks DB: *BRS Biochemistry,* 2nd ed. Baltimore, Williams & Wilkins, 1994, p 24.)

- Glycine and proline are "helix busters." They disrupt the secondary structure of proteins.
- Cysteine can bind with other cysteines via an oxidative reaction to form a disulfide bond (R-S-S-R).

b. Protein Structures

- **Primary structure** refers to the specific amino acid sequence.
- **Secondary structure** refers to the presence of regularly repeated three-dimensional structures, notably α-helices (especially in membrane-spanning proteins) and β-pleated sheets (e.g., keratin).
- **Tertiary structure** is the total three-dimensional structure of a peptide.
- **Quaternary structure** is the structure of a protein made of multiple peptides, such as the four subunits of hemoglobin that bind around the central iron ion.

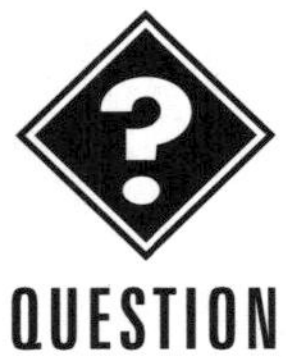

QUESTION

Which amino acids are likely to be found inside the protein?

ANSWER

As mentioned previously, the hydrophobic amino acids are most likely to be found inside the protein because this part of the protein is not usually in contact with water. The hydrophobic amino acids are valine, leucine, isoleucine, phenylalanine, and methionine (see Table 2-14).

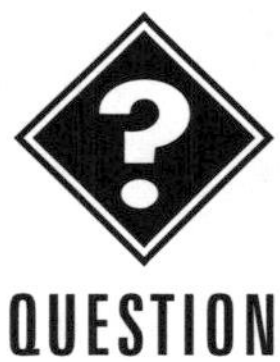

QUESTION

Which amino acids are likely to be found on the outside of the protein?

ANSWER

Along the same lines as the preceding answer, any amino acid other than hydrophobic amino acids are likely to be found on the outside of the protein, which is in contact with the hydrophilic, aqueous intra- and extracellular fluid.

Which amino acids are most likely to be found at the active site of the protein?

QUESTION

Which amino acids are present at the active site depends on the chemical nature of the substrate. If the substrate is positively charged, an acidic amino acid that is negatively charged (R–COO^-), such as aspartate or glutamate, would most likely be found in the active site, attracting and holding onto the cationic substrate. Conversely, a negatively charged substrate would require the presence of a positively charged basic amino acid (R-NH_3^+), such as lysine, arginine, or histidine, to form an electrostatic interaction with the anionic substrate.

ANSWER

Which amino acids are most likely to be found on histone proteins?

QUESTION

Positively charged amino acids (e.g., lysine, arginine, histidine) found in histone proteins enable them to interact with DNA, which is highly negatively charged because of its phosphate backbone.

ANSWER

11 AUTONOMIC NERVOUS SYSTEM

a. Sympathetic Nervous System

Often referred to as the **"fight or flight"** component, the sympathetic nervous system ganglia are all in the spinal cord; therefore, the preganglionic neurons are short and the postganglionic neurons are long (Figure 2-46). The sympathetic nervous system increases energy expenditure, accelerates the heart, increases metabolism, inhibits digestion, and diverts blood flow to the muscles. In other words, it prepares the organism for action (Table 2-15).

b. Parasympathetic Nervous System

Often called the **"rest and digest"** component, the parasympathetic nervous system ganglia are near the organs themselves; that is, the preganglionic neurons are long and postganglionic neurons are short (see Figure 2-46). The parasympathetic nervous system enhances activities that conserve and gain energy, such as decreased heart rate, decreased metabolism, increased digestive action, and increased blood flow to the gut (see Table 2-15 for further details).

TABLE 2-15. System function and response

System Function	Sympathetic Response	Parasympathetic Response
Heart rate and contractility	Increased	Decreased
Pupillary reaction	Dilation	Constriction
Respiratory system action	Bronchodilation	Bronchoconstriction
Gastrointestinal motility and blood flow	Decreased	Increased
Glycogen metabolism	Breakdown (catabolic)	Synthesis (anabolic)
Blood flow to skeletal muscle	Increased	Decreased

c. Renin–Angiotensin System (Figure 2-47)

1. **Angiotensinogen** is a plasma protein that is produced by the liver. The majority of plasma proteins are produced by the liver, with the exception of antibodies, which are produced by specialized B cells (plasma cells).

2. **Renin** is produced by the juxtaglomerular cells of the kidney. These cells are also responsible for producing erythropoietin, which stimulates the bone marrow to produce red blood cells.

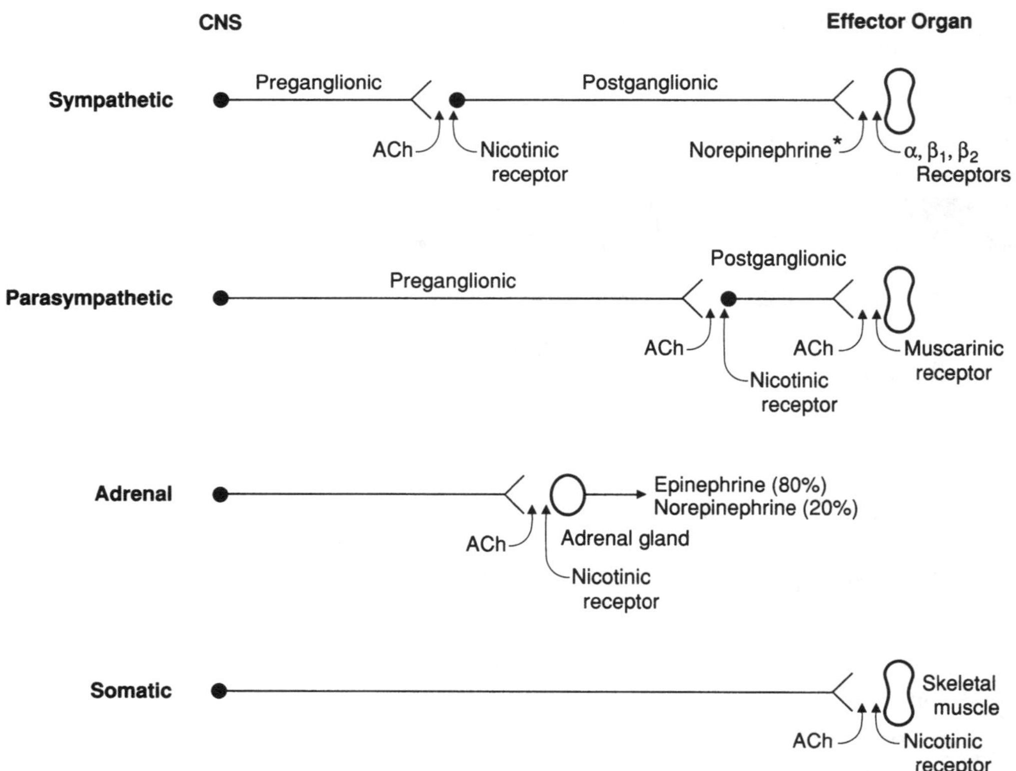

Figure 2-46. Organization of the autonomic nervous system. (Reprinted with permission from Marks DB: *BRS Biochemistry*, 2nd ed. Baltimore, Williams & Wilkins, 1994, p 30.)

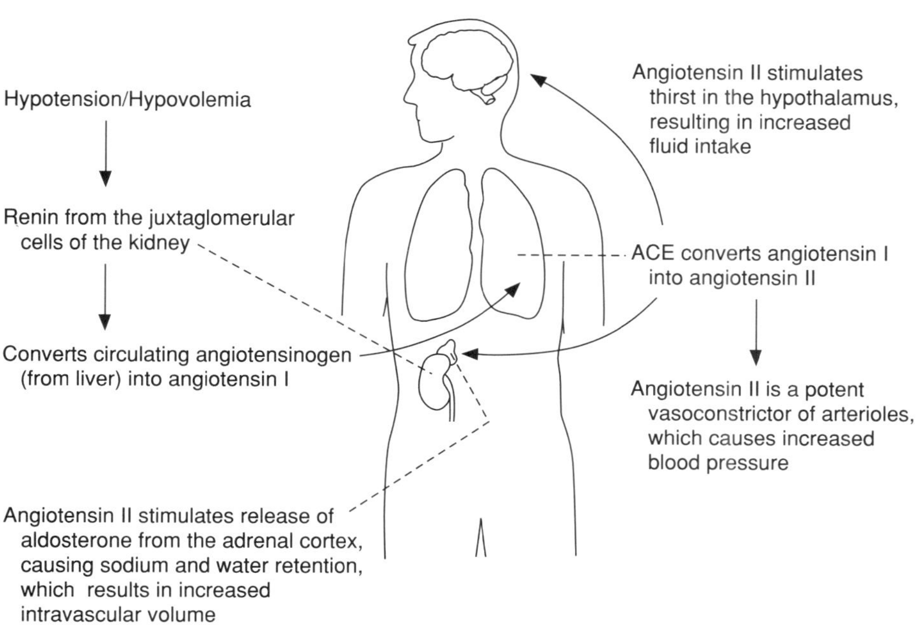

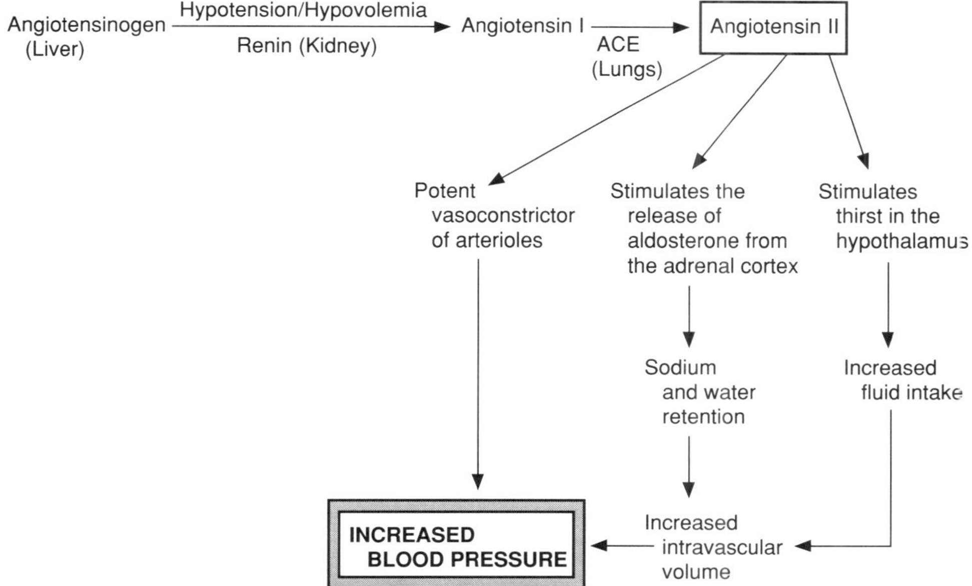

Figure 2-47. Renin–angiotensin system. *(A)* Physiologic responses to hypotension/hypovolemia. *(B)* Flow chart showing the mechanisms by which the renin–angiotensin system increases blood pressure. *ACE* = angiotensin-converting enzyme.

d. Baroreceptor Reflex

This phenomenon occurs when hypotension (low blood pressure) stimulates the release of catecholamines (epinephrine and norepinephrine) from the sympathetic nervous system, causing an increased heart rate and thus preserving cardiac output. Remember:

$$\text{Cardiac output} = \text{heart rate} \times \text{stroke volume}$$

e. Cardiovascular

responses to exercise and hemorrhage (Tables 2-16 and 2-17).

TABLE 2-16. Summary of effects of exercise

Heart rate	↑↑	
Stroke volume	↑	
Cardiac output	↑↑	
Arterial pressure	↑	(slight)
Pulse pressure	↑	(due to increased stroke volume)
TPR	↓↓	(due to vasodilation of skeletal muscle beds)
AV O_2 difference	↑↑	(due to increased O_2 consumption)

AV = atrioventricular; *TPR* = total peripheral resistance.
Reprinted with permission from Costanzo LS: *BRS Physiology*, Baltimore, Williams & Wilkins, 1995, p 94.

TABLE 2-17. Summary of responses to hemorrhage

Heart rate	↑	
TPR	↑	
Contractility	↑	
Unstressed volume	↓	(↑ stressed volume)
Renin	↑	
Angiotensin II	↑	
Aldosterone	↑	
Circulating epinephrine and norepinephrine	↑	
ADH	↑	

ADH = antidiuretic hormone; *TPR* = total peripheral resistance.
Reprinted with permission from Costanzo LS: *BRS Physiology*, Baltimore, Williams & Wilkins, 1995, p 94.

12 ENDOCRINE REGULATION

Peptide hormones are released more quickly and have more rapid effects than steroid hormones, making them the more rapid response system. It takes longer for steroid hormones to act because they work at the level of DNA, subsequently altering protein synthesis, thereby creating a longer term effect.

a. Peptide hormones

(Table 2-18) cannot pass through the cell membrane because they are hydrophobic (the largely lipid plasma membrane is lipophilic). Instead, these hormones **bind to cell membrane receptors** and activate **second messengers.** The best-known second messenger is **cyclic AMP** (cAMP) [Figure 2-48]. A peptide hormone binds to a receptor, which then activates a **G protein,** which in turn activates the enzyme

TABLE 2-18. Hormones and their functions

Hormone	Type of Hormone	Source	Target	Function
ADH (vasopressin)	Peptide	Hypothalamus (synthesis) Posterior pituitary (secretion)	Kidney (collecting ducts)	Stimulates retention of water in the kidney by increasing the collecting ducts' permeability to water. Alcohol consumption suppresses ADH secretion.
Oxytocin	Peptide	Hypothalamus (synthesis) Posterior pituitary (secretion)	Uterus	Induces labor by stimulating uterine contraction; also causes breast to eject milk
***Growth hormone (GH)**	Protein	Anterior pituitary	Many organs, including liver	Stimulates growth of bone, muscle, and other tissues
Adrenocortico-tropic hormone (ACTH)	Protein	Anterior pituitary	Adrenal cortex	Stimulates synthesis and secretion of cortisol from adrenal cortex
Luteinizing hormone (LH)	Protein	Anterior pituitary	Testes Ovaries	Stimulates secretion of testosterone by testes Stimulates ovulation and formation of corpus luteum in females
Follicle stimulating hormone (FSH)	Protein	Anterior pituitary	Testes Ovaries	Stimulates spermatogenesis in testes Stimulates development of follicle in ovary
Thyroid stimulating hormone (TSH)	Protein	Anterior pituitary	Thyroid	Stimulates production and secretion of thyroid hormones
Prolactin	Protein	Anterior pituitary	Breast tissue	Stimulates production of milk by breast
T_3 and thyroxine (T_4)	Peptide (cytoplasmic receptor)	Thyroid gland	Many organs, including heart	Increases basal metabolic activity in many tissues and sensitizes heart to catecholamines
Parathyroid hormone (PTH)	Peptide	Parathyroid gland	Bone, kidney	Increases serum calcium by causing bone resorption (stimulates osteoclast activity) and decreases calcium excretion by the kidney
Calcitonin	Peptide	Thyroid gland	Bone	Decreases serum calcium by causing calcium deposition in bone. Also inhibits bone resorption by inhibiting osteoclasts
***Glucocorticoids (e.g., cortisol)**	Steroid	Adrenal cortex	Many organs, including liver	Many effects, including increasing blood glucose levels and reducing inflammatory response
Mineralocorti-coids (e.g., aldosterone)	Steroid	Adrenal cortex	Kidney (distal tubule)	Causes sodium and water retention by distal tubule, as well as potassium excretion into the urine
***Catecholamines (e.g., epinephrine and norepinephrine)**	Peptides	Adrenal medulla	Many organs, including heart, pupil, and blood vessels	Coordinates all fight-or-flight responses (see Table 2-15)

Continued

TABLE 2-18. Hormones and their functions—Cont.

Hormone	Type of Hormone	Source	Target	Function
†Insulin (antagonistic to glucagon, cortisol, epinephrine, norepinephrine & GH)	Protein	Beta-islet cells of pancreas	Many organs, including liver, muscle, and adipose tissue	Anabolic hormone: decreases blood glucose by stimulating synthesis of glycogen from glucagon; also stimulates lipid and protein biosynthesis
***Glucagon (antagonistic to insulin)**	Protein	Alpha-islet cells of pancreas	Many organs, including liver, muscle, and adipose tissue	Catabolic hormone: increases blood glucose by stimulating glycogen breakdown; also stimulates lipid and protein degradation
Progesterone	Steroid	Ovaries Placenta	Endometrium	Promotes growth of uterine endometrium and decreases contraction of myometrium
Estrogen	Steroid	Ovaries Placenta	Many organs, including bone	Many functions, including maintaining bone density and developing and maintaining female secondary sexual characteristics
Testosterone	Steroid	Leydig cells of testes	Many organs	Many functions, including development of muscle and bone and development of male secondary sexual characteristics

*These hormones are hyperglycemic (raise blood glucose concentrations); they stimulate both the breakdown of glycogen to glucose and gluconeogenesis (anabolic).
†Insulin is the only hypoglycemic hormone (lowers blood glucose concentrations); it stimulates the synthesis of glycogen from glucose and inhibits glycogenolysis (catabolic).

adenylate cyclase. Adenylate cyclase subsequently catalyzes the transformation of ATP to cAMP. An increase in intracellular cAMP can then mediate many different biologic reactions, often via the action of a **cAMP-dependent protein kinase** that phosphorylates proteins and changes their activity.

b. Steroid hormones

(see Table 2-18; Figures 2-49 and 2-50) are much more hydrophobic and therefore can pass right through the plasma membrane. They reach the nucleus and **bind to nuclear receptors, cytoplasmic receptors,** or both. These steroid receptors, once bound to the incoming steroid hormone, then bind to DNA and directly influence DNA transcription. This occurs via binding to specific enhancer sequences that recognize the steroid receptor's DNA-binding domain.

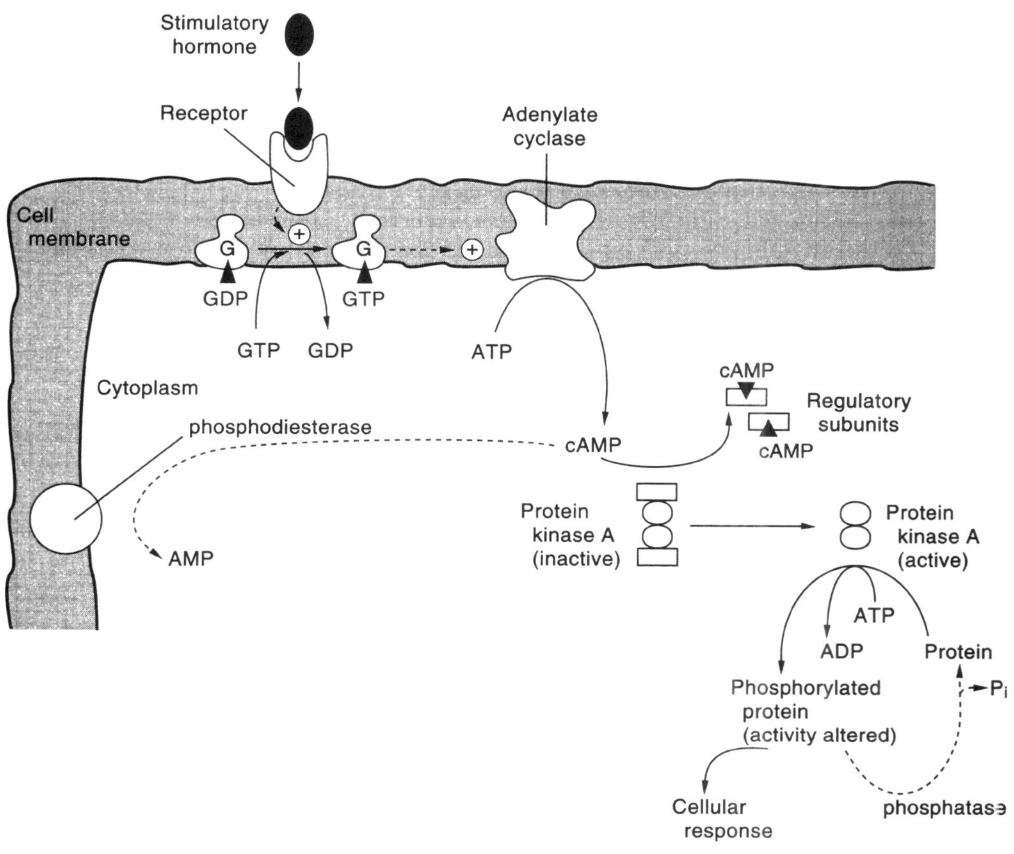

Figure 2-48. The production and action of cyclic AMP (cAMP). *G* = G protein. G proteins function when GTP is bound; ○ = free catalytic subunits; ▭ = regulatory subunits of protein kinase A; ⊕ = stimulates. (Reprinted with permission from Marks DB: *BRS Biochemistry*, 2nd ed. Baltimore, Williams & Wilkins, 1994, p 280.)

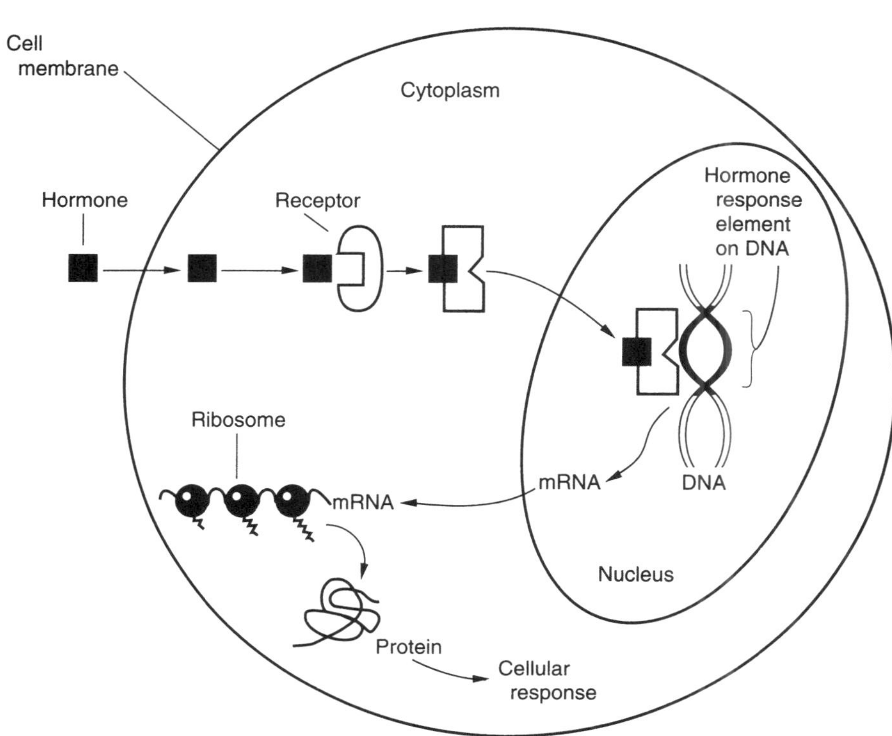

Figure 2-49. The mechanism of action of hormones of the steroid–thyroid family. (Reprinted with permission from Marks DB: *BRS Biochemistry*, 2nd ed. Baltimore, Williams & Wilkins, 1994, p 284.)

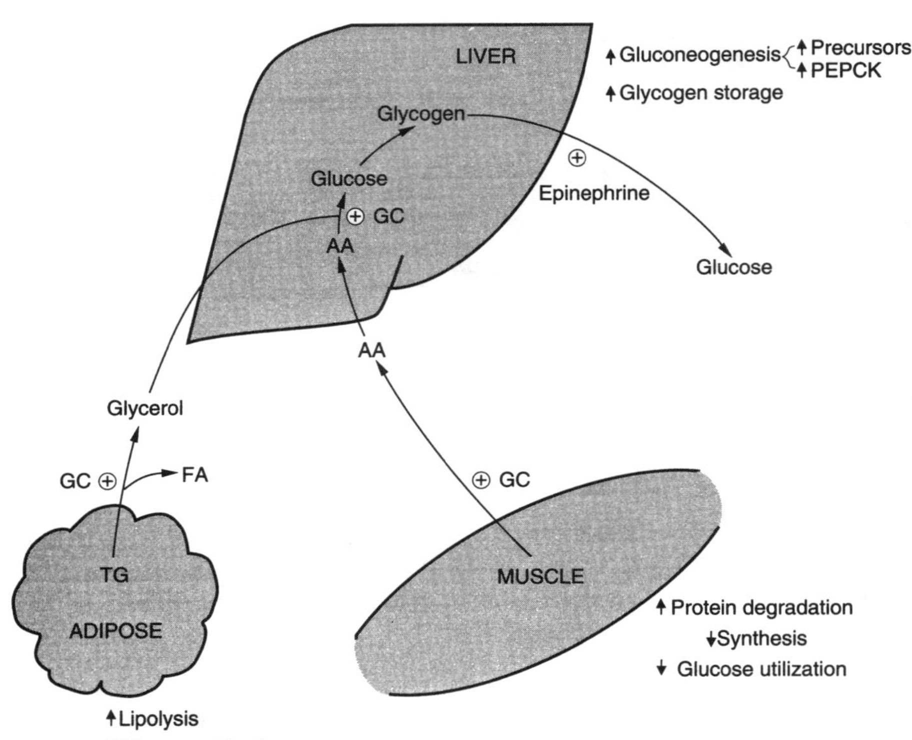

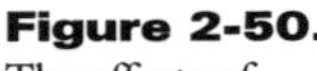
Figure 2-50.
The effects of glucocorticoids *(GC)* and epinephrine on fuel metabolism. (Reprinted with permission from Marks DB: *BRS Biochemistry,* 2nd ed. Baltimore, Williams & Wilkins, 1994, p 288.)

13 DIGESTION AND ABSORPTION

The bulleted items and Tables 2-19 and 2-20 outline nutrient transport for digestion and absorption.

The liver is the first organ to receive digested food from protein- and lipid-rich blood and lymph.

- Fatty acids and triacylglycerides (TAGs) are packaged as chylomicrons and are carried in the lacteals (part of the lymphatic system), which drain into the liver.
- All other materials, such as carbohydrates and amino acids, are carried in the bloodstream via the portal circulation to the liver.
- Therefore, digested food **first** makes its way to the liver, which distributes its metabolites to all the other organs of the body.
- Bile salts emulsify fats and fat-soluble vitamins (vitamins A, D, E, and K) and are absorbed in the ileum of the small intestine (Figures 2-51 and 2-52). Therefore, if a good portion of the ileum is resected for any reason (e.g., cancer), this loss of absorptive surface could result in fat malabsorption, resulting in deficiencies of fat-soluble vitamins (A, D, E, K) as well as vitamin B_{12} deficiency (because vitamin B_{12} is bound to intrinsic factors and absorbed in the ileum), which causes anemia and neurologic problems.
- **Cholesterol** is the precursor of bile and steroid hormones.

TABLE 2-19. Digestion and absorption of carbohydrates, proteins, and lipids

Nutrient	Enzyme	Site of Production	Site of Function	Function
Carbohydrates	Ptyalin (Salivary amylase)	Salivary glands	Mouth	Starch → maltose
	Lactase	Intestinal glands	Small intestine	Lactose → glucose and galactose
	Sucrase	Intestinal glands	Small intestine	Sucrose → glucose and fructose
	Maltase	Intestinal glands	Small intestine	Maltose → 2 glucose
	Pancreatic amylase	Pancreas	Small intestine	Starch → maltose
Proteins	Pepsin†	Gastric glands	Stomach	Hydrolyzes certain peptide bonds
	Trypsin†	Pancreas	Small intestine	Hydrolyzes certain peptide bonds
	Chymotrypsin†	Pancreas	Small intestine	Hydrolyzes peptide bonds
	Carboxypeptidase	Pancreas	Small intestine	Hydrolyzes terminal carboxyl peptide bond
	Aminopeptidase	Intestinal glands	Small intestine	Hydrolyzes terminal amino peptide bond
	Dipeptidases (e.g., lactase)	Intestinal glands	Small intestine	Hydrolyzes amino acid pairs
	Enteropeptidase	Intestinal glands	Small intestine	Converts trypsinogen to trypsin
Lipids	Bile*	Liver	Small intestine	Emulsifies fats and fat-soluble vitamins (A, D, E, K)
	Lipase	Pancreas	Small intestine	Hydrolyzes lipids

*Bile is not an enzyme. It emulsifies fat globules, making it easier for pancreatic lipase to break down fats.
†Trypsin, pepsin, and chymotrypsin are initially secreted in their inactive forms (known as zymogens: trypsinogen, pepsinogen, and chymotrypsinogen), then activated when they reach their final site of action. Trypsinogen is converted to trypsin by the enzyme enteropeptidase; trypsin in turn converts chymotrypsinogen to chymotrypsin and activates aminopeptidases and carboxypeptidases. Pepsinogen is converted to pepsin by the low pH of the stomach.

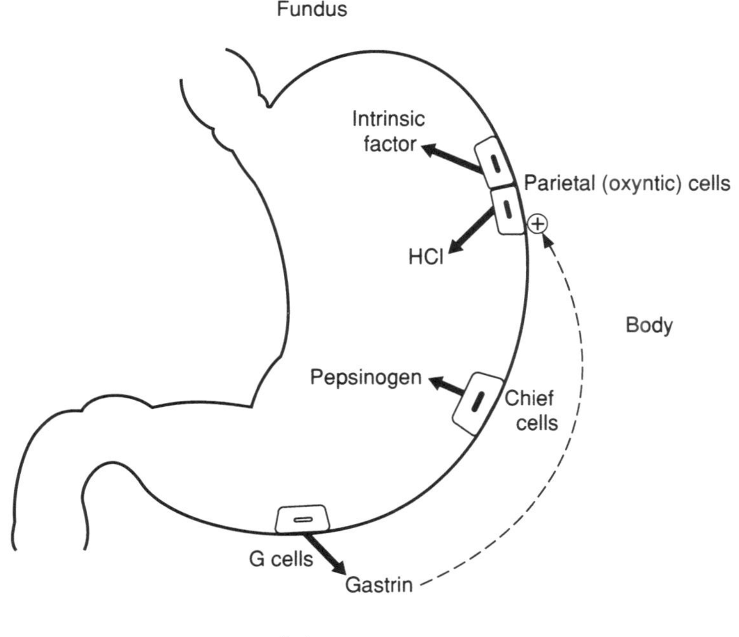

Figure 2-51. Gastric cell types and their functions. (Reprinted with permission from Costanzo LS: *BRS Physiology*, Baltimore, Williams & Wilkins, 1995, p 193.)

TABLE 2-20. Summary of digestion and absorption

Nutrient	Digestion	Site of Absorption	Mechanism of Absorption
Carbohydrates	To monosaccharides (glucose, galactose, fructose)	Small intestine	Na^+-dependent cotransport (glucose, galactose) Facilitated diffusion (fructose)
Proteins	To amino acids, dipeptides, tripeptides	Small intestine	Na^+-dependent cotransport
Lipids	To fatty acids, monoglycerides, cholesterol	Small intestine	Micelles form with bile salts in intestinal lumen Diffusion of fatty acids, monoglycerides, and cholesterol into cell Reesterification in the cell to triglycerides and phospholipids Chylomicrons form in the cell (requires apoprotein) and are transferred to lymph
Fat-soluble vitamins		Small intestine	Micelles with bile salts
Water-soluble vitamins		Small intestine	Na^+-dependent cotransport
Vitamin B_{12}		Ileum of small intestine	Intrinsic factor
Bile acids		Ileum of small intestine	Na^+-dependent cotransport; recirculated back to the liver
Ca^{2+}		Small intestine	Vitamin D-dependent Ca^{2+}-binding protein
Fe^{2+}	Fe^{3+} is reduced to Fe^{2+}	Small intestine	Binds to apoferritin in the cell Circulates in blood bound to transferrin

Reprinted with permission from Costanzo LS: *BRS Physiology*, Baltimore, Williams & Wilkins, 1995, p 200.

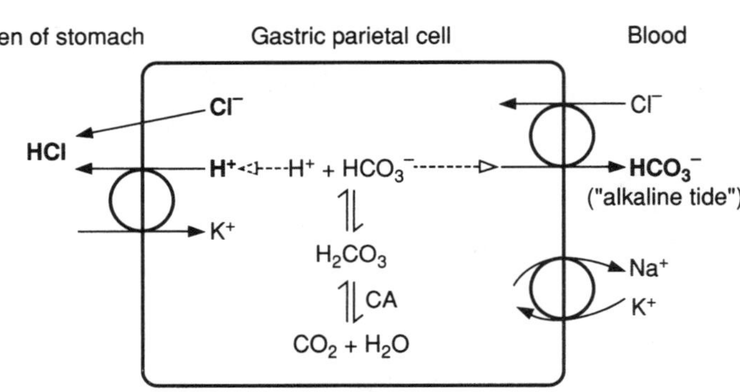

Figure 2-52.
Simplified mechanism of secretion of H^+ by gastric parietal cells. (Reprinted with permission from Costanzo LS: *BRS Physiology*, Baltimore, Williams & Wilkins, 1995, p 193.)

14 THE PANCREAS AND THE LIVER

a. Pancreas

The pancreas is both an exocrine and an endocrine organ.

- Exocrine functions of the pancreas include secretion of digestive enzymes (e.g., pancreatic lipase, amylase, trypsin, chymotrypsin).
- Endocrine functions of the pancreas include hormone secretion of insulin and glucagon.

Because the pancreas is both an endocrine and exocrine organ, destruction of the pancreas (e.g., chronic pancreatitis) can result in diabetes mellitus (endocrine dysfunction) as well as protein, fat, and vitamin A, D, E, and K (fat-soluble vitamins) malabsorption (exocrine dysfunction).

b. Liver

The liver performs many functions:

- Synthesis of bile from cholesterol
- Synthesis of many serum proteins, including albumin and clotting factors
- Drug detoxification (e.g., alcohol)
- Storage of vitamins and minerals (e.g., vitamin A, vitamin E, vitamin B_{12}, iron, copper)

It is a major site of metabolism, including:

- **Gluconeogenesis** (conversion of lactic acid to glucose)
- **Interconversion of carbohydrates**
- **Fatty acid degradation,** resulting in the formation of ketone bodies

Along with the spleen, the liver contributes to the destruction and removal of old erythrocytes and circulating immune complexes. The **Kupffer cells,** specialized macrophages in the liver, remove old erythrocytes and circulating immune complexes from the bloodstream.

15 OXYGEN TRANSPORT IN THE BODY

a. Hemoglobin

Hemoglobin is a complex polypeptide protein that has four subunits (two α subunits and two β subunits) bonded together around an iron ion. This complex can reversibly bind four oxygen molecules, making it an ideal oxygen carrier for the circulatory system, allowing the red blood cells to deliver oxygen to all the cells in the organism. The structure of hemoglobin is highly conserved through evolution, and hemoglobin protein sequence homology can be used to delineate recency of ancestry. In addition, fetal hemoglobin (expressed before birth) is slightly different from adult hemoglobin (expressed after birth).

Fetal hemoglobin has an increased oxygen affinity because it cannot bind 2,3-BPG as well as adult hemoglobin can.

Figure 2-53 charts how well hemoglobin within the blood binds to oxygen. The sigmoid-shaped oxygen dissociation curve increases rapidly at moderate oxygen partial tension (oxygen concentration) and increases more slowly at very low or very high oxygen partial tension. This is caused by positive cooperativity as a result of interaction between the four protein subunits in the hemoglobin molecule.

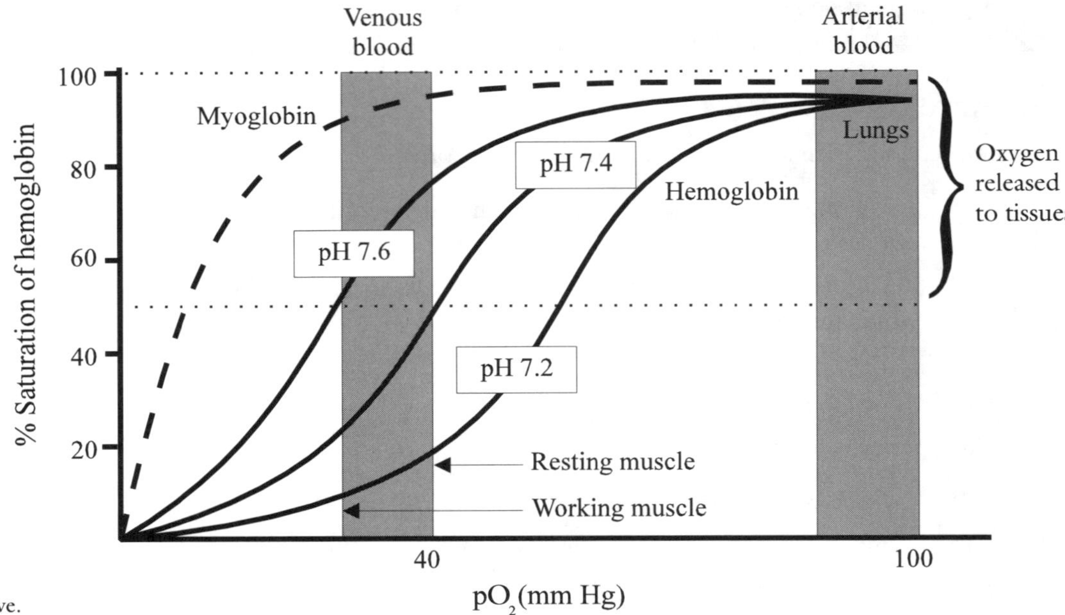

Figure 2-53. Hemoglobin and myoglobin binding curve.

b. Myoglobin

Myoglobin is similar to hemoglobin found in mammalian muscular tissue; but unlike hemoglobin, myoglobin binds oxygen at very low oxygen tensions (see Figure 2-53). Active muscle cells can deplete the surroundings of oxygen and therefore depend on myoglobin for oxygen transport and supply. In a low oxygen tension environment, hemoglobin has very little oxygen to release to the muscle. Diving mammals, who must adapt to an oxygen-depleted environment, have a high blood concentration of myoglobin, which allows them to transport oxygen in their blood even when oxygen levels drop to dramatic lows. And unlike hemoglobin, which is composed of four subunits, myoglobin is a single subunit protein that exhibits a hyperbolic- (not sigmoid) shaped oxygen dissociation curve (see Figure 2-53).

c. High Altitudes

People physiologically adapt to living at high altitudes by producing more erythrocytes, a process that takes approximately 30 days and is stimulated by erythropoietin.

At high altitudes, the low atmospheric pressure means that the partial pressure of oxygen is lower than the pressure at sea level. This means that we move **along the curve** to a lower partial oxygen pressure (pO_2), corresponding to a lower oxygen saturation in the blood, which causes you to feel tired at high altitudes. However, if you live at high altitudes, your cardiovascular system cannot adapt quickly to this higher altitude because it takes approximately 1 month to make new red blood cells. However, other species can produce a hemoglobin molecule with a higher affinity for oxygen under conditions of low atmospheric pressure, which means that the oxygen dissociation curve shifts to the left (for a given pO_2 there is a higher oxygen saturation percent) owing to the increased ability of hemoglobin to bind and transport oxygen in oxygen-depleted surroundings. At high altitudes, the body initially compensates for the lower oxygen saturation in the blood by producing 2,3-BPG (see Section E, Bohr effect).

d. Erythropoietin

Red blood cell production is stimulated by the hormone erythropoietin, which is made by the juxtaglomerular cells of the kidney (also the site of renin production) in response to a low arterial blood oxygen concentration (PaO_2). These cells sense the low concentration of oxygen in the blood under certain conditions (e.g., high altitudes, lung disease) and secrete erythropoietin, which stimulates the bone marrow to make more oxygen-carrying red blood cells.

e. Bohr Effect

Higher temperatures, acidity, and 2,3-BPG increase the unloading of oxygen from red blood cells.

Under different environmental conditions, the hemoglobin dissociation curve changes through a phenomenon called the **Bohr effect,** which shifts the oxygen curve to the right. The Bohr effect occurs during conditions of acidity, elevated carbon dioxide levels, increased temperature, and increased 2,3-BPG. When these conditions occur, cells can increase their ability to pick up oxygen from the blood by increasing the extracellular pH of its surroundings, which induces hemoglobin to give up more of its oxygen to the oxygen-starved cells in the peripheral tissues. The Bohr effect is important because it facilitates the offloading and delivery of oxygen to the hypoxic target organs (leg muscles anaerobically producing lactic acid). At high altitudes, the body produces 2,3-BPG, which facilitates the unloading of oxygen to its target organs. This action compensates for the lack of oxygen content in the air.

16 BIOLOGY OF MUSCLE CONTRACTION

a. Muscle Types

- **Skeletal muscle** is voluntary and includes the muscles of the hand, arm, and leg. This muscle has striations.
- **Smooth muscle** is involuntary. It is found in the stomach, arteries, bladder, and other locations.
- **Cardiac muscle** is involuntary and is found exclusively in the heart. It has striations and intercalated disks.

b. Sarcoplasmic reticulum

is a specialized type of smooth endoplasmic reticulum found in all types of muscle cells that sequester calcium ions. The sarcoplasmic reticulum has voltage-dependent calcium channels. When the muscle cell is depolarized by neuronal stimulation, these channels open, releasing calcium ions from the sarcoplasmic reticulum and stimulating muscle contraction.

c. Actin

is a globular protein with one heavy and two light chains (the light chains wrap around the heavy chain). The head of the actin molecule can bind to myosin and make muscles contract in the presence of ATP by forming **cross-bridges**. The actin molecules make up the thin filaments of the sarcomere.

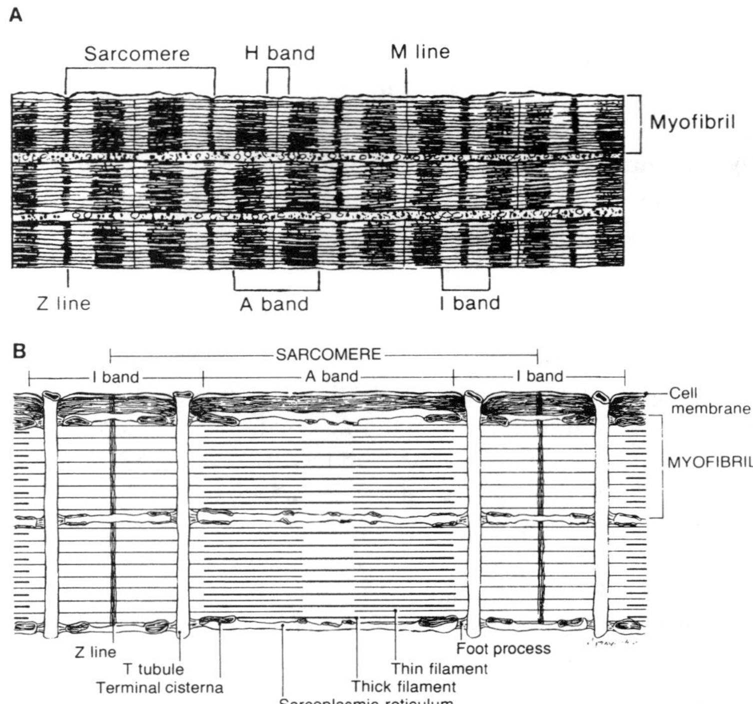

Figure 2-54. The sarcomere: thick and thin filaments. *A band* = length of one thick filament (does not change during contraction); *H band* = area with only thick filaments (shortens during contraction); *I band* = area with only thin filaments (shortens during contraction); *thick band* = myosin filaments; *thin band* = actin filaments; *Z line* = distance of one sarcomere (shortens during contraction). (Reprinted with permission from Bullock J, Boyle J, Wang MB: *NMS Physiology*, 2nd ed. Baltimore, Williams & Wilkins, 1991, p 29.)

d. Myosin

is a type of globular protein that provides a binding site for the head group of the actin molecule. It forms the thick filaments of the sarcomere (Figure 2-54).

17 BONE GROWTH AND REMODELING

a. Osteoclasts

are cells responsible for bone resorption (breakdown of bone).

b. Osteoblasts

are cells responsible for laying down the protein matrix of the bone. The process of bone formation is coupled with bone resorption; that is, osteoclasts and osteoblast actions must be coordinated.

c. Parathyroid hormone (PTH)

Osteoclasts have been found to have estrogen receptors on their surface; when activated by estrogen, these receptors inhibit osteoclast activity and therefore prevent osteoporosis.

stimulates the breakdown of bone, mostly through the action of osteocytes and some osteoclasts (Figure 2-55 and Table 2-21). This resorption of bone increases serum calcium levels (in fact, PTH is the most important regulator of serum calcium levels) by decreasing the amount of calcium that is secreted by the kidneys. PTH also stimulates the renal enzyme that converts vitamin D to a more active form that can increase intestinal uptake of calcium and renal reabsorption of calcium. PTH stimulates the renal excretion of serum phosphate (a product of bone resorption) into the urine.

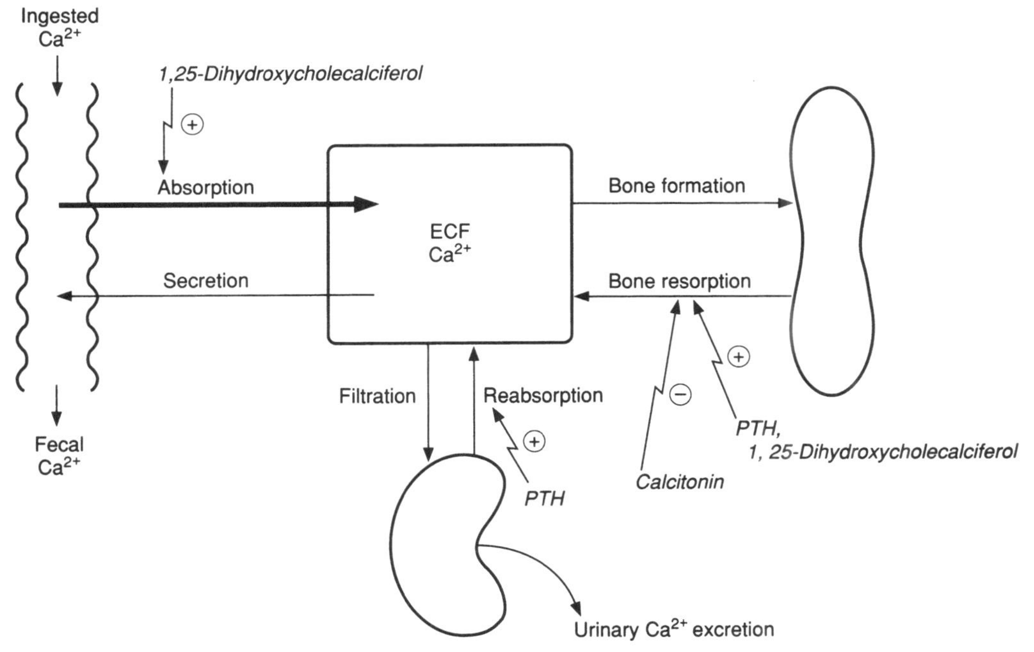

Figure 2-55. Hormonal regulation of Ca^{2+} metabolism. *ECF* = extracellular fluid; *PTH* = parathyroid hormone. (Reprinted with permission from Costanzo LS: *BRS Physiology*, Baltimore, Williams & Wilkins, 1995, p 236.)

TABLE 2-21. Summary of hormones regulating Ca^{2+}

	PTH	Vitamin D	Calcitonin
Stimulus for secretion	↓ serum [Ca^{2+}]	↓ serum [Ca^{2+}] ↑ PTH ↓ serum [phosphate]	↑ serum [Ca^{2+}]
Actions on:			
Bone	↑ resorption	↑ resorption	↓ resorption
Kidney	↓ P reabsorption (↑ urinary cyclic AMP) ↑ Ca^{2+} reabsorption	↑ P reabsorption ↑ Ca^{2+} reabsorptior	
Intestine	↑ Ca^{2+} absorption (via vitamin D)	↑ Ca^{2+} absorption (vitamin D-dependent Ca^{2+}-binding protein) ↑ P absorption	
Overall effect on:			
Serum [Ca^{2+}]	↑	↑	↓
Serum [phosphate]	↓	↑	

P = phosphate; PTH = parathyroid
Reprinted with permission from Costanzo LS: *BRS Physiology*, Baltimore, Williams & Wilkins, 1995, p 235.

d. Calcitonin

decreases serum calcium levels by stimulating the movement of serum calcium into bone, resulting in bone formation. It also inhibits osteoclastic activity, thereby inhibiting bone resorption. Calcitonin increases the level of calcium and phosphorus in urinary excretion. Levels of calcitonin may rise right after a meal in response to gastrin secretion.

e. Vitamin D

in the active form causes increased absorption of dietary calcium from the gut as well as increased calcium reabsorption in the kidney. Vitamin D is ingested in an inactive form that is modified in the liver and in the kidney, which activate this molecule's ability to influence the digestive system and renal system. PTH acts on the kidney to stimulate conversion of vitamin D into its active form.

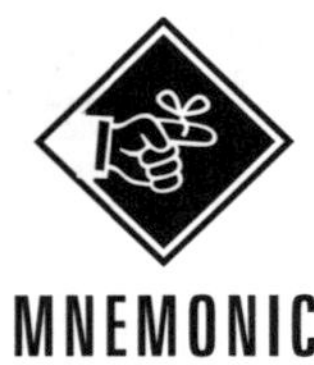

MNEMONIC

"Calcitonin" rhymes with **"bone in"** (it puts calcium in bone by stimulating osteoblasts and inhibiting osteoclasts). Osteo**b**lasts are **b**uilders whereas osteo**c**lasts are **c**arvers of bone.

18 IMMUNOLOGY

a. Antigen

is any foreign molecule that stimulates a specific immune response; proteins are the most effective antigens.

B cells are responsible for humoral (antibody-mediated) immunity, whereas T cells are responsible for cell-mediated immunity.

b. Antibody

is an immunoglobulin that is secreted by plasma cells and can function as an antibody receptor on a B cell. The antibody reacts with the antigen (which originally stimulated its production) to neutralize it or make it more ingestible for phagocytic cells; this process is called **opsonization**.

1. An **immunoglobulin** (Figure 2-56) is another term for antibody; the five classes of immunoglobulins are as follows:

   (a) **IgA,** monomer or dimer. IgA is the antibody secreted by the cells of the different "tracts" (e.g., gastrointestinal, respiratory). IgA is found in bodily secretions and is the major antibody given to infants in their mothers' milk right after birth. Secretory IgA protects the mucous membranes from bacteria and viruses. It binds with antigens, and the invading antigen–antibody complex is then swept from the body's mucosal surfaces.

   (b) **IgM,** pentamer. IgM is the largest and most abundant immunoglobulin produced during the initial (primary) response to an invading microorganism. It is restricted to the bloodstream, where it

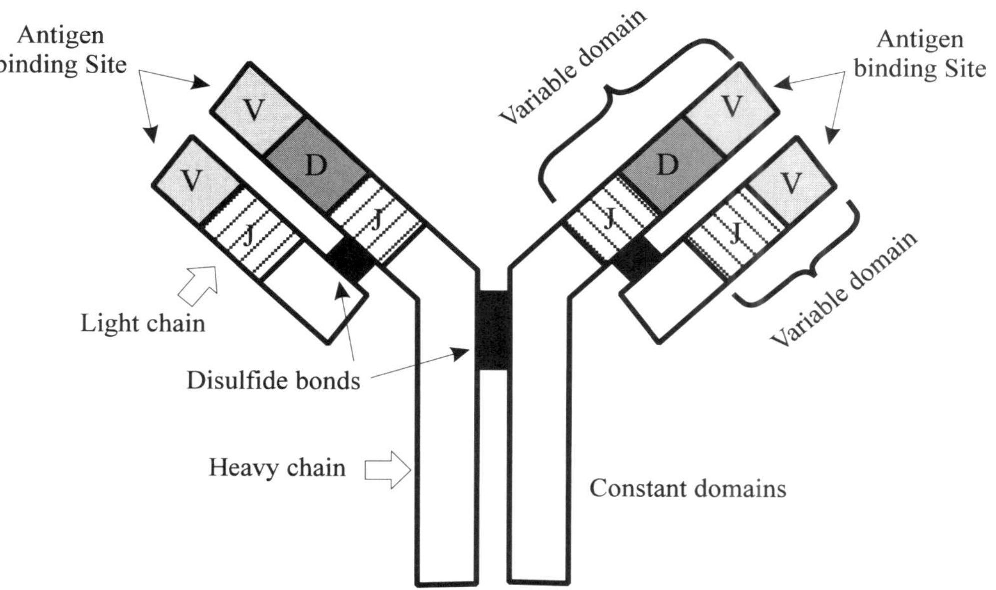

Figure 2-56. Immunoglobulin.

can cluster (agglutinate) antigens and activate the complement immune response.

(c) **IgG,** monomer. IgG is the most abundant of the circulating antibodies (IgG constitutes more than 80% of all antibodies in the plasma). It can cross capillary molecules easily and can also cross the placenta. An organism must be exposed to high antigen concentrations before a specific IgG is made. These antibodies destroy cells by activating complement. IgG is produced in the secondary immune response to a previously encountered antigen.

(d) **IgD,** monomer. IgD is bound to the plasma membrane of B cells. It is the primary antigen receptor of immunocompetent B cells.

(e) **IgE,** monomer. This antibody is associated with some of the body's immune responses and is found in increased numbers in people with allergies. IgE can bind to mast cells, which release histamine as part of the allergic response.

2. Antibodies, like any other protein, are encoded by genes. **Antibody diversity** is generated by the recombination and rearrangement of DNA segments coding for the V, D, and J segments of the heavy chain as well as the V and J segments of the light chain (i.e., gene shuffling) [Figure 2-57]. When a specific combination is produced to generate an antibody that is capable of binding to a specific antigen, interleukins as well as other cytokines are produced by helper T cells, which stimulate the differentiation of B cells to antibody-producing plasma cells.

c. Bone marrow

is the source of all blood cells and other blood components (e.g., red blood cells, B and T lymphocytes, platelets, macrophages, neutrophils). Radiation can kill the rapidly dividing stem cells of the bone marrow, thereby causing immunosuppression (by killing lymphocyte precursors) and anemia (by killing red blood cell precursors).

Bone marrow precursors mature into red blood cells, white blood cells (granulocytes and lymphocytes), and platelets, and are very sensitive to radiation.

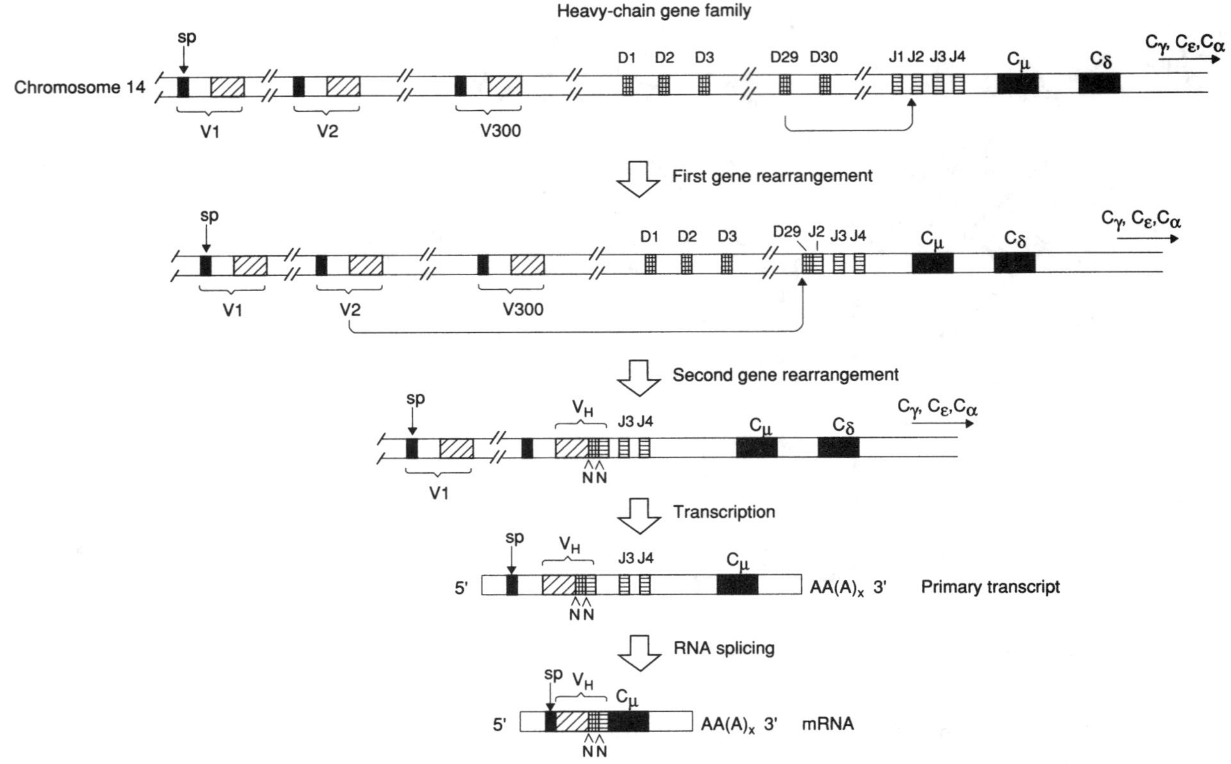

Figure 2-57.
Example of the formation of a heavy-chain (*H*) immunoglobulin-gene. Heavy-chain formation takes place by joining a partial variable region of the heavy chain *(V_H)*, the diversity region (*D*), and the joining region of the heavy chain *(J_H)*, which requires two DNA rearrangements. In the *first gene rearrangement,* one of about thirty D segments *(D29)* is moved immediately upstream of one of four J_H genes *(J2)*. The ***second gene rearrangement*** moves one of about three hundred partial V_H genes *(V2)* immediately upstream of the newly joined D and J segments *(D29-J2)* to form a complete exon that codes for the V_H domain. During these DNA rearrangements, up to 30 nucleotides *(N)* may be added between the V and D and the D and J segments by terminal deoxynucleotidyl transferase. Splicing of the primary transcript of this newly formed heavy-chain gene removes the intron between the V_H exon and the exon that codes for the constant *(C)* domain for immunoglobulin M (i.e., C_u). The intron between the exon that codes for the signal peptide *(sp)* and the V_H exon is also removed by splicing. Translation of this messenger RNA *(mRNA)* is directed to the endoplasmic reticulum (*ER*). (Reprinted with permission from Davidson VL, Sittman DB: *NMS Biochemistry,* 3rd ed. Baltimore, Williams & Wilkins, 1994, p 273.)

19 EMBRYOLOGICAL DERIVATIVES OF GERM LAYERS (TABLE 2-22)

TABLE 2-22. Embryological derivatives of germ layers

Primary Germ Layer	Resulting Structures
Ectoderm	Skin (including hair and the lens of the eye) Nervous system (including the brain, spinal cord, and peripheral nerves)
Endoderm	Epithelium of digestive system (e.g., esophagus, stomach, intestines) Epithelium of respiratory system (e.g., trachea, lungs) Inner linings of visceral organs (e.g., lungs, heart, gastrointestinal tract)
Mesoderm	Everything else (e.g., muscles, bone, kidneys, gonads, spleen, and the circulatory system)

20 MEIOSIS VERSUS MITOSIS

Figure 2-58 shows the process of mitosis and meiosis.

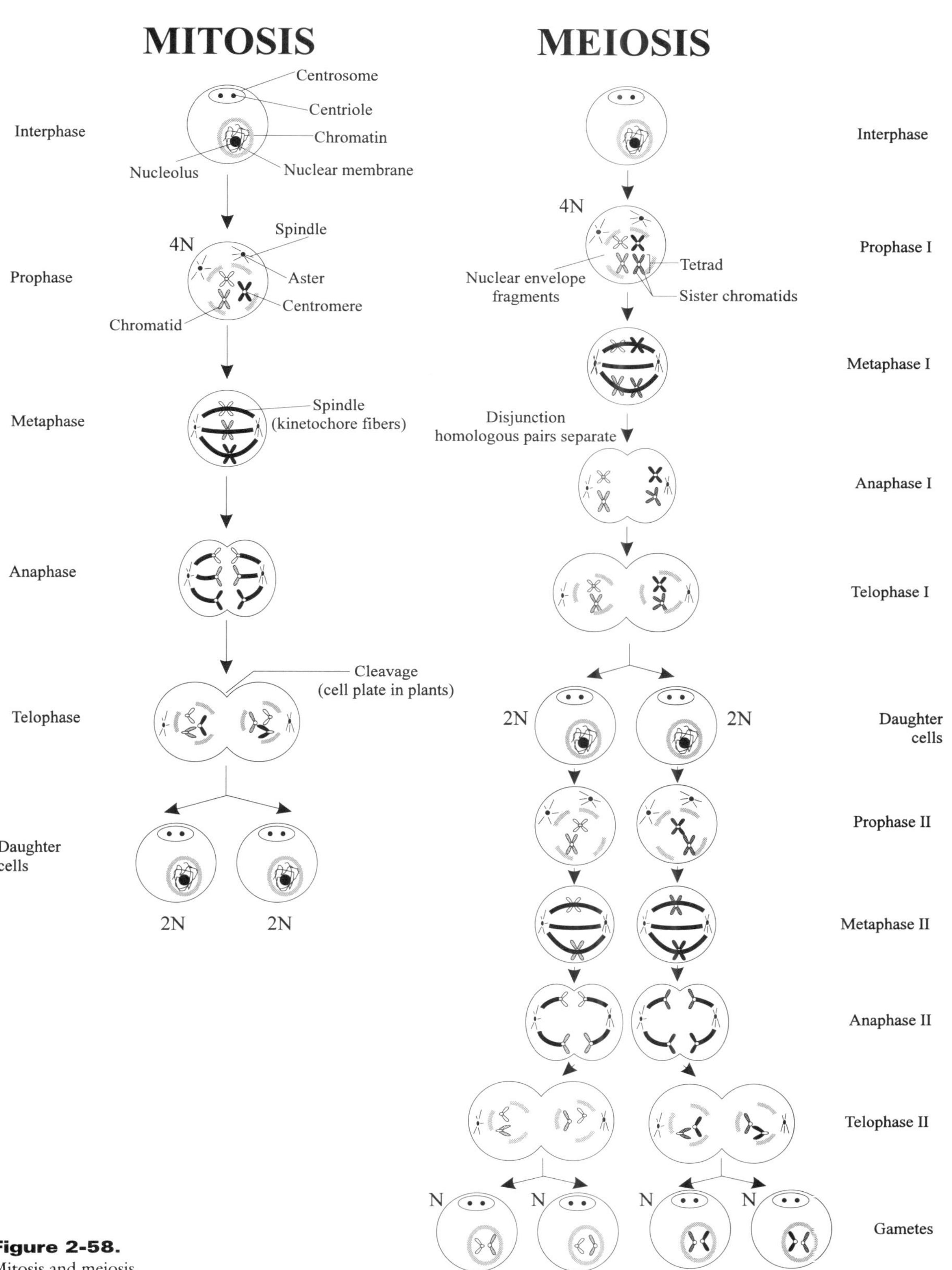

Figure 2-58.
Mitosis and meiosis.

PART III

mcat review books

A Word About Review Books ...

THIS SECTION PROVIDES information on the MCAT books and study aids that are currently available. Each publication has been assigned a letter grade based on factors such as content, usability, and price. These ratings reflect the experience and opinions of many premed students who used the resources listed below. We invite your opinions and ratings (see How to Contribute).

Rating

A = Excellent resource—a "must-buy"
B = Very good—gets the job done
C = Adequate, but better resources are available

For each book we provide the address and phone number for ordering directly from the publisher. We also give you the scoop on the books with overviews and "bottom line" evaluations. Before you buy anything, make sure you think about your available study time and your willingness to study independently.

A+ MCAT PRACTICE TEST II AND MCAT PRACTICE ITEMS

Association of American Medical Colleges
Membership and Publication Orders
2450 N Street, NW
Washington, DC 20037-1126
(202) 828-0416

Price: $20.00 plus $5.00 shipping and handling
Format: Test
Questions: 220; 685
Pages: 290 in two booklets

The *MCAT Practice Test II* (220 questions) is a reprint of the actual April 1991 MCAT. The *MCAT Practice Items* consists of 265 verbal reasoning and 420 physical/biological sciences passage-based questions, with letter answers only. These two booklets were written by the Association of American Medical Colleges (AAMC), the same friendly folks who bring you the MCAT. Therefore, the questions in these booklets have the same format, level of difficulty, detail, and content emphasis as do the MCAT questions.

Bottom line. This set of booklets is a "must-buy" and very high yield. The *MCAT Practice Test II* is a useful full-length diagnostic exam to take a week or two before the actual MCAT under simulated testing conditions. The *MCAT Practice Items* are an excellent source of practice questions and are indispensable as a study aid. Student experience shows that the topics and content covered in these questions are a very reliable predictor of many topics that are tested on the actual MCAT.

A+ MCAT PRACTICE TEST III

Association of American Medical Colleges
Membership and Publication Orders
2450 N Street, NW
Washington, DC 20037-1126
(202) 828-0416

Price: $20.00 plus $5.00 shipping and handling

Format: Test

Questions: 220

Pages: 134

Like the *MCAT Practice Tests I* and *II,* this book contains sample test questions from past MCATs. Many of these questions are from the 1994 MCAT. There is one full-length practice test, which includes a writing sample. Letter answers are provided only for multiple-choice components of the test. However, sample essays with a critique are included for evaluating the writing sample.

Bottom line. As the most recent of the released AAMC MCAT practice tests, *MCAT Practice Test III* does the best job of simulating the current MCAT. This is also a "must-buy"!

A MCAT STUDENT MANUAL AND MCAT PRACTICE TEST I

Association of American Medical Colleges
Membership and Publication Orders
2450 N Street, NW
Washington, DC 20037-1126
(202) 828-0416

Price: $20.00 plus $5.00 shipping and handling

Format: Review/Test

Questions: 315

Pages: 210 in two booklets

The *MCAT Student Manual* includes an orientation chapter written by the test makers. This section covers the format and content of the MCAT as well as a description of how the MCAT is scored. In addition, the *MCAT Student Manual* includes fairly descriptive and detailed outline of the science content on the MCAT, which can be used as a study guideline. According to the AAMC, this outline contains all the possible topics that are tested on the MCAT. Finally, the *MCAT Student Manual* provides 95 sample questions with answers and detailed explanations.

The *MCAT Practice Test I* is a full-length diagnostic exam with 220 questions. This practice test was used as the template for the new MCAT examination. Unfortunately, there are no explanations to the answers (only letter answers are given).

Bottom line. You should purchase these books. The *MCAT Student Manual* is the official (although probably not the best) guide to the MCAT. In addition, it provides useful study and test-taking advice. The practice test may be a little dated, but it is still close to the real MCAT. Consider using this as a diagnostic tool as you begin your MCAT preparation.

A– ARCO'S MCAT SUPERCOURSE®/ARCO SAMPLE EXAMS

Macmillan General Reference
15 Columbus Circle
New York, NY 10023
(800) 428-5331

Price: $35.00 plus $3.50 shipping and handling ($13.95 for *ARCO Sample Exams* only)

Format: Review/Test

Questions: 900+ (657 in three full-length tests plus many review questions)

Pages: 700

ISBN: 0671848445 and 0135444381 for the *Sample Exams*

ARCO's MCAT SuperCourse® contains comprehensive reviews of the four components of the MCAT. Each review unit is peppered with plenty of practice problems and is followed by a full-length subject-specific practice test with answers and explanations. Three full-length practice exams are also sold separately as *ARCO MCAT Sample Exams.* For this reason, do not buy the *ARCO Sample Exams* if you plan on purchasing the *SuperCourse®*. In addition to a basic orientation to the MCAT, *SuperCourse®* also provides a brief description of medical school and residency training.

Bottom line. This book offers a solid combination of content review and practice tests. It has a strong, comprehensive review of all the major scientific topics covered on the MCAT. The balanced reviews have plenty of questions, key words, and useful charts. The physical sciences and biology chapters are excellent. The organic chemistry section may be the only weak area. Learning is reinforced with subject-specific practice tests. The verbal reasoning unit is pretty good, but be aware that the verbal reasoning passages are easier than those on the actual MCAT. Three full-length practice exams offer students ample opportunity to simulate the MCAT. Explanations to the practice tests are very helpful. However, physical and biological science passages are shorter, and the questions that follow focus more on a student's discrete knowledge of each subject than on the ability to identify key concepts.

A– COLUMBIA REVIEW'S INTENSIVE PREPARATION FOR THE MCAT

Williams & Wilkins
351 W. Camden Street
Baltimore, MD 21201-2436
(800) 638-0672

Price: $43.95 plus shipping and handling
Format: Review/Test
Questions: 829
Pages: 825
ISBN: 0683010271

Kaplan and Princeton Review are not the only test preparation companies coming out with MCAT books. Columbia Review weighs in with its own review text that features a comprehensive review of biology, organic chemistry, physics, and inorganic chemistry in an outline format. Students can test their progress with the sample problems throughout the text and with the 120 passage-based questions at the end of each science section. Also, two practice verbal reasoning tests and a full-length sample MCAT are included. In addition, a 40-page guide introduces the student to the MCAT and provides study and test-taking strategies.

Bottom line. Columbia Review does an excellent job of providing the reader with a concise yet exhaustive content review in under 850 pages. This book can be read in less than six weeks. The easy-to-read outline format provides appropriate coverage of MCAT topics without straying into needless detail. The text is complemented by useful and easy-to-understand tables and diagrams. Practice MCAT-style questions at the end of each section closely simulate the real MCAT. Helpful explanations to the practice questions are a major plus. Use this book in conjunction with the AAMC *MCAT Practice Tests* to round out a balanced MCAT preparation regimen.

A− FLOWERS & SILVER MCAT 97–PRINCETON REVIEW

Random House
400 Hahn Road
Westminster, MD 21157
(800) 733-3000

Price: $50.00 plus $4.00 shipping and handling
Format: Review
Questions: 250+
Pages: 1045
ISBN: 0679771069

Just when you thought MCAT books couldn't get any bigger, Flowers does it again, first with the Betz MCAT guide (with which he is no longer affiliated) and now with the new *Flowers & Silver MCAT 97* from Princeton Review. Flowers took only one thing when leaving Betz for Princeton: a propensity for big books and the wacky numbering system (remember topic 16.1.4.2.4?). The Flowers book provides a systematic review of all science topics that are likely to be tested on the MCAT. Each topic is reinforced with problems scattered throughout the text and with a simulated MCAT passage with answers and explanations at the end of each chapter. In addition, basic mathematics, quantitative skills, and reading comprehension are reviewed.

Bottom line. Despite its intimidating size, the Flowers book is easy to read and understand. It covers both the fundamentals and the necessary finer points. It emphasizes concepts and avoids needless detail. Occasionally, the verbosity of the text slows the reader. The text is filled with quality diagrams, figures, and tables. Surprisingly, this book has only a modest, but well written, number of practice passages. You can supplement this book with simulated practice exams (e.g., AAMC *MCAT Practice Tests*). If you use this book, budget at least 2 to 3 months and plenty of stamina to get through it. It'll be a marathon.

B+ KAPLAN MCAT ALL-IN-ONE

Bantam Doubleday Dell Publishing Group
1540 Broadway
New York, NY 10036
(800) 323-9872

Price: $34.95 plus $2.50 shipping and handling
Format: Orientation/review/test
Questions: 328 (two thirds in book and one third on disk)
Pages: 275
ISBN: 038531633X

This new book (updated in 1996) is a comprehensive but not overwhelming source of information for the entire medical school application process. It is divided into four components: medical school admissions, which provides basic information and strategy for developing an application, deciding where to apply, and interviewing; MCAT review, which briefly discusses general strategies and test-taking mentality and briefly provides section-specific reviews containing strategies and sample questions with answers and explanations; a full-length practice MCAT exam; and a half-length practice exam on disk (Mac/Win). Plugs for Kaplan's test preparation course are scattered throughout the text.

Bottom line. *Kaplan MCAT All-in-One* has a little something for everyone, but not everything for anybody. The admissions section is useful, but short compared with other books that dedicate themselves entirely to the admissions process. The MCAT advice is also helpful and humorous but not complete. The full-length practice MCAT with answers and explanations (yes!) is an adequate simulation of the real MCAT. The computer software is user friendly and provides questions with answers and explanations, data about your performance, and information on your test-taking habits. This book can get you started, but it won't take you all the way.

B THE BEST TEST PREPARATION FOR THE MCAT

Research and Education Association (REA)
61 Ethel Road West
Piscataway, NJ 08854
(908) 819-8880

Price: $42.95 plus $7.75 shipping and handling

Format: Review/Test

Questions: 1320 in six full-length practice tests plus content-review questions

Pages: 1002

ISBN: 0878918728

Best Test Preparation for the MCAT consists of comprehensive reviews of the subjects tested on the MCAT (including a mathematics review), along with six full-length practice tests with detailed explanations. The reviews are organized to parallel the content outline in the *MCAT Student Manual.* The introduction to this book discusses MCAT format and scoring and general test-taking strategies.

Bottom line. If you are looking for a book with lots of practice tests for your dollar, then REA's book is for you. The REA examination questions are similar in both format and difficulty to those that are on the MCAT. Plus, detailed explanations to every question answer are provided (bravo!).

The science reviews are comprehensive and well written, but they may not be adequate as a primary review source for some students. The authors include review questions at the end of each section. The directory of medical schools that REA includes is probably useless, because you should already have the AAMC's *1996–97 Medical School Admission Requirements.*

B FLOWERS & SILVER ANNOTATED PRACTICE MCATs

Random House
400 Hahn Road
Westminster, MD 21157
(800) 733-3000

Price: $20.00 plus $2.00 shipping and handling. $34.95 with diagnostic test disk plus $4.00 shipping and handling

Format: Orientation/Test

Questions: 219 in the book and 657 on the disk

Pages: 210

ISBN: 0679771271, 0679771050 (CD-Rom), 0679771042 (3.5″ disk)

Formerly titled *Cracking the MCAT,* this book is divided into three sections: orientation, diagnostic test, and diagnostic explanations to answers. The orientation section provides information about the format of the MCAT. Following the Princeton Review philosophy (i.e., the "Joe Bloggs approach"), the suggested strategies are based on intuition and common sense. The full-length diagnostic test includes detailed explanations to answers. The optional disk (Mac/Win) provides two additional sample tests. These tests are timed, generating scores automatically and providing letter answers after each question you finish.

Bottom line. The one full-length diagnostic test is a dandy. It is one of the best non-AAMC practice tests available. Reprinting the questions next to the answers and explanations is a great idea! Use the diagnostic test as one of your final practice exams (along with the AAMC

MCAT Practice Test III). The additional tests on disk provide great practice, but they have no explanations. The orientation guide to the MCAT is not very helpful. It is less of a strategy guide to the MCAT than a lead-in for Princeton Review's test preparation course.

B– A COMPLETE PREPARATION FOR THE MCAT: THE BETZ GUIDE

Williams & Wilkins
351 W. Camden Street
Baltimore, MD 21201
(800) 638-0672

Price: $49.50 plus $4.00 shipping and handling
Format: Review
Questions: 1250 (140 MCAT-type questions)
Pages: 800
ISBN: 0941406296

Formerly called *Flowers' Guide to the MCAT,* the hefty *Betz Guide* boasts a massive and detailed science review. Of the book's 1250 questions, 1100 are content-review questions that appear at the end of each chapter, testing your knowledge of the specific information presented. *A Complete Preparation for the MCAT* does not contain any full-length exams; there are only 140 MCAT-style questions that appear as a series of passage-based questions in the final part of the book. However, the book is currently undergoing a major revision.

Bottom line. Students have used the *Betz Guide* since the time of Hippocrates, but this publication's age now shows. As the MCAT has evolved, more material has been added to this book without removing some of the outdated material. As a result, this book is far too detailed in many places, especially in its review of the physical and biological sciences. The content review questions at the end of each chapter are not typical of those asked on the actual MCAT. The mathematics review is only helpful to those who have a very weak math background. The new edition due in 1996 promises to address these problems.

Some students who use this book never complete it. Therefore, we recommend this book only for the highly motivated student who starts MCAT preparation at least 4 to 6 months in advance.

B– CADUCEUS SOFTWARE FOR THE MCAT

Scientia
657A Summerville Avenue
Summerville, MA 02143
(800) 453-4725

Price: $135.00 plus $5.00 shipping and handling
Format: Review
Questions: 800 (non-MCAT style)
ISBN: 1885727003 (Mac), 1885727011 (PC), 1885727046 (CD-ROM)

Caduceus MCAT Review is a multimedia software review that covers physics, biology, inorganic chemistry, and organic chemistry. The software presents lessons that cover basic science topics. Concepts are brought to life with color animation clips and illustrations. You can test your comprehension of the topic with the click of a button at anytime. Convenient options include the ability to print out topics on paper and to place "bookmarkers" at topics that need extra attention.

Bottom line. Caduceus is a well-written piece of software that may be better suited for remedial science review than for MCAT preparation. The visuals and animated graphics are outstanding, and the user interface is very intuitive. However, the questions are not MCAT style and do not test your ability to apply information under test conditions. Use this tool only in conjunction with other review books.

C+ BARRON'S HOW TO PREPARE FOR THE MCAT

Barron's Educational Series, Inc.
250 Wireless Boulevard
Hauppauge, NY 11788
(516) 434-3311

Price: $12.95 plus $3.75 shipping and handling

Format: Review/Test

Questions: 900

Pages: 475

ISBN: 0812046463

This book is divided into three major sections. The first section is an overview of the actual MCAT and includes a rough conversion of raw scores to MCAT scores. The second section provides a review of physics, biological science, and chemistry. The third section consists of four full-length practice exams with answers and explanations.

Bottom line. Barron may do a decent job with its SAT and Achievement Test reviews, but its MCAT review book is disappointing. The introduction is somewhat helpful, but the book goes downhill from there. The science review sections suffer from the Goldilocks syndrome: sometimes too much information (i.e., biology section), sometimes too little (i.e., chemistry section), but never just right. In addition, the book tends to emphasize reactions and mathematics without adequately covering concepts that will be tested.

The four exams in this book do not accurately reflect the style of the MCAT. The verbal reasoning passages are significantly longer than MCAT passages (which are deliberately condensed by the AAMC). On the other hand, the biological and physical sciences passages are too short and the physical science questions are too math-oriented (i.e., "plug and chug"). Although this book is inexpensive, saving $30 on a comprehensive review book should not be a factor when MCAT scores are on the line.

C+ BETZ MCAT DIAGNOSTIC EXAMS (PRACTICE TESTS 4, 5, AND 6)

Williams & Wilkins
351 W. Camden Street
Baltimore, MD 21201
(800) 638-0672

Price: $29.95 each plus $4.00 shipping and handling

Format: Test

Questions: 219

Pages: 78

ISBN: 0941406644

These publications each contain a full-length MCAT simulation that you mail for free computer scoring and analysis. The test itself does a good job of simulating the form and content of the current MCAT. An answer key without explanations is included in a sealed envelope. After taking the practice exam under test conditions, you send the scoring sheet and writing sample essays to the computer-scoring center. Two weeks later, you receive a 6-page report that identifies your weaknesses in MCAT skills and content. You can opt for express scoring service (3 working days), but it will cost you another $20.

Bottom line. The report is of limited benefit. You receive grades for your writing samples, but no written critique. To fully understand the report, you must have *A Complete Preparation for the MCAT: The Betz Guide* to explain the problem-solving skills that are evaluated. The lack of explanations for questions that are answered incorrectly also limits the usefulness of the analysis. Finally, the 2-week turnaround for scoring and analysis is too long to be useful; by the time you get your results, your preparation may be at a completely different stage. In addition, you may have forgotten most of that exam. Express scoring service, which costs you extra money, is a must if you want to maximize the utility of the report.

C AAMC MCAT VIDEOTAPE: PREPARING FOR THE MCAT

Association of American Medical Colleges
Membership and Publication Orders
2450 N Street, NW
Washington, DC 20037-1126
(202) 828-0416

Price: $12.00 plus $7.00 shipping and handling

Format: Orientation

This 25-minute video produced by the AAMC is an introduction to preparation for the MCAT. It briefly discusses the format and structure of the MCAT, and it provides basic study tips and suggestions.

Bottom line. Unfortunately, this videotape plays like a long "infomercial" for the MCAT. All of the information provided is similar to that in the *MCAT Student Manual,* but without all of the useful tips. If you're a student who likes a little visual motivation to get started, you may want to borrow the video if your university or career center has a copy.

C– FUTURE TEST MCAT

National Learning Corporation
212 Michael Drive
Syosset, NY 11791
(516) 921-8888

Price: $69.95 plus $6.00 shipping and handling

Format: Review

Questions: 3500+

ISBN: 0837394279

Future Test MCAT is an interactive, self-paced software program available for both Macintosh® and MS-DOS computers. The review covers basic science information in six sections through terms with definitions and questions with answers. The final exam can be custom tailored to contain a specific number of questions under specific time restrictions. Most questions on the exams are direct recall. There are neither problem-solving nor passage-based questions. After quizzes and exams, *Future Test* provides a "report card" to track your progress.
Bottom line. The material is very basic, almost remedial, and the questions, which are not in an MCAT style, provide little practice for the actual exam. In addition, there is no organization of the topics covered. This software review is expensive and has minimal preparatory value for the MCAT.

C– NEW RUDMAN'S QUESTIONS AND ANSWERS ON THE MCAT

National Learning Corporation
212 Michael Drive
Syosset, NY 11791
(516) 921-8888

Price: $23.95 plus $6.00 shipping and handling

Format: Test

Questions: 2000+

Pages: 375

ISBN: 0837350115

This book contains about 2000 MCAT-style questions with letter answers only. Explanations are not provided. It includes a brief 5-page introduction about study and test-taking strategies.

Bottom line. This book has many poorly written, outdated questions. Most questions are not passaged-based and test knowledge rather than the ability to interpret and apply concepts. Also, the questions are not organized in the standard MCAT format. In addition, the production quality is mediocre; it looks like it was created on a typewriter. Don't spend too much time on these practice questions.

C– MCAT PREPARATION GUIDE

University Press of Kentucky
663 South Limestone Street
Lexington, KY 40508-4008
(800) 839-6855

Price: $15.95 plus $3.00 shipping and handling

Format: Strategy guide

Questions: None

Pages: 137

ISBN: 0813108470

The *MCAT Preparation Guide* is a book designed to be a companion to the AAMC *MCAT Student Manual.* The guide first discusses some basic test-taking techniques for the multiple-choice sections of the exam and offers a stepwise strategy to approaching the writing sample. It then provides a series of tables keyed to *MCAT Practice Test I.* These tables help you identify your weaknesses in each section of *MCAT Practice Test I.*

Bottom line. *MCAT Preparation Guide* has an interesting approach to the MCAT, but it doesn't provide much MCAT "enlightenment." Because the analysis is derived from only one practice test (as opposed to an analysis based on performance over several practice tests, which can reveal true trends and weaknesses). This book neither reviews any topics nor provides explanations to questions. In addition, many of the test-taking strategies and techniques are too basic and nonspecific.

PART IV

mcat course reviews

A Word About Review Courses ...

MORE AND MORE students preparing for the MCAT are turning to review courses. The competition for admission to medical school has heated up, and students are looking to others for help in getting an edge on the MCAT. Commercial review courses can be effective in organizing material and guiding a student who is overwhelmed by the "MCAT experience." In response to the demand, new review courses continue to appear. Ten years ago, there were only one or two choices, but now there are at least five, and the list grows annually. The two national courses are Kaplan and Princeton Review. Berkeley Review, Columbia Review, and Hyperlearning are regional review courses that are largely based on the West Coast.

Although many students are satisfied with their review course experience, commercial review courses are not a "magic pill" for everyone's MCAT woes. Many cited cost as a major issue; at around $800 for each review course, the concern is well founded. One comment of almost all students, regardless of the review course they took, was that studying for the MCAT didn't become quite as "easy, fast, and fun" as promised. Some students said that they had fallen for the advertising hype.

On the next few pages is some information on the major review courses. This information is intended to supplement your decision on whether to attend a review course. The following are some tips for evaluating a review course:

- Ask yourself what you are looking for in an MCAT review course (e.g., discipline, organization, specialized study materials) and if the time and financial commitments are worth it.
- Find out if the course fits your schedule and your style of learning. Some classes are offered on evenings and weekends.
- Tour the learning center, look at the review materials, ask about the qualifications of the instructors, and sit in on a class if possible.
- Talk to friends and classmates who have taken review courses.

Don't expect that paying for a review course will motivate you to study. Only *you* can motivate yourself to study! We welcome your opinions on review courses, so we can include evaluations in future editions. Note that review courses evolve continually and prices, format, and availability are subject to change. We recommend that you call each commercial review course for the latest available information.

National Review Courses

THE PRINCETON REVIEW

2315 Broadway, 3rd Floor
New York, NY 10024-4332
(800) 995-5565

Cost: $895–$1000 (regional costs may vary; ask about financial aid)

Classroom hours: 60

Class size: 8–12 students per instructor

Length: 9 weeks

The Princeton Review course emphasizes strategies and concepts rather than memorization techniques. The course extends approximately 9 weeks, with 2 to 3 meetings per week, each lasting about 3 hours. Its small classes are interactive. The Princeton Review course includes four full-length proctored mock MCAT exams (8 hours each), and up to 20 hours of free tutoring is available. The course includes the Caduceus software, a package for MCAT science review (see Part III). The Princeton Review course also provides study materials to use at home, including a comprehensive science review covering biology, organic chemistry, physics, and general chemistry and three sample MCAT exams.

STANLEY H. KAPLAN EDUCATIONAL CENTER

810 Seventh Avenue, 26th Floor
New York, NY 10019
(800) KAP-TEST or (800) 527-8378

Cost: $895 (regional costs may vary; ask about financial aid and alumni and campus discounts)

Classroom hours: Approximately 40–50

Class size: 10–30 students per instructor

Length: 4–6 weeks

The three parts of the Kaplan course are (1) review books, (2) classroom sessions, and (3) the test-and-tape laboratory. The course's home study materials include four review books covering the MCAT sciences and a fifth review book that focuses on the verbal reasoning and writing sample sections. Approximately 10 classroom sessions (4 hours each) are given over a 4- to 6-week period. The class format may vary from center to center. Students take a simulated MCAT at the beginning and at the end of the course. During the course, students are given homework assignments and go over problems with the instructor during classroom sessions. Classroom sessions are also available on tape for student review and makeup. Kaplan's test-and-tape laboratory has flexible hours, including evenings and weekends. Kaplan instructors include premeds who have scored well (95th percentile or better) on the MCAT as well as graduate and medical students.

Regional Review Courses

THE BERKELEY REVIEW

P.O. Box 40140
Berkeley, CA 94704
(510) 843-8378
(800) 622-8827

Cost: $795 (work–study program available for students with financial need)

Hours: 110

Class size: 25 students per classroom

Length: 15 weeks

The Berkeley Review course provides an intensive four-point system that includes classroom instruction, comprehensive review books, practice exams, and office hours. The classroom instruction is for 15 weeks, four 2-hour sessions per week. These sessions usually involve thorough discussion of MCAT passages and questions, including multiple timesaving strategies and approaches. Writing techniques for the essay are also reviewed. Comprehensive review books that cover all MCAT subjects and six full-length exams that students may complete at home are provided. Office hours are offered for the verbal reasoning section, including one-on-one essay and verbal reasoning analysis. Practice exams test each of the various subjects, one full-length exam assesses progress in the middle of the course, and two mirror the MCAT under simulated conditions at the very end of the course.

THE COLUMBIA REVIEW

220 Madison Avenue
San Francisco, CA 94134
(800) 300-PREP
(415) 337-2009

Cost: $695 (regional costs may vary; ask about financial aid and alumni and campus discounts)

Classroom hours: 100+

Class size: 20–25 per classroom

Length: 9–13 weeks

The Columbia Review course emphasizes concepts and passage analysis rather than memorization of facts. It is an intensive MCAT preparation course that combines many hours of class time with lots of practice tests and home-study materials. A home-study program is available at a cost of $325 for students who do not live near a Columbia Review center. The course for the April MCAT begins in January and lasts 13 weeks (meeting twice weekly plus small-group study sessions). The course for the August MCAT begins in June and lasts 9 weeks (meeting three times weekly plus small-group study sessions). The course reviews first the physical sciences, then the biological sciences, with a review of verbal reasoning and essay writing throughout. The course includes more than 50 hours of small-group study sessions devoted to helping students who have specific weaknesses. Individual tutorials are also available. The Columbia Review supplements its 100 hours of classroom instruction with an array of home-study materials, including review notes, formula sheets, problem sets, practice tests, and all MCAT material currently available from the AAMC. The primary course instructors are academic MDs, MD–PhD candidates, and graduate students.

HYPERLEARNING

8950 Villa La Jolla Drive, Suite 1131
La Jolla, CA 92037
(619) 455-1000, (800) MD-BOUND, (714) 725-9192

Cost: \$825 (regional costs may vary; ask about financial aid and alumni and campus discounts)

Hours: 100+

Class size: 20–25 students per classroom

Length: 12 weeks

The Hyperlearning course attempts to give a comprehensive and intensive review of the verbal, physics, chemistry, and biological areas of the MCAT. This review course offers approximately 2000 pages of review material and more than 100 hours of instruction, with 4 days of classes weekly (over 40 classes total). Each class lasts for 2½ hours. Each week, one section each of physics, chemistry, biology, and verbal reasoning is covered. There are 8 weeks of general chemistry followed by 4 weeks of organic chemistry. There are 12 weeks of biology and 10 weeks of physics. Additional passages are provided for students to use during their home study. The verbal section focuses on verbal reasoning and the writing sample essay. Hyperlearning also offers students additional one-on-one help with essay writing for an additional \$50. The course offers five full-length practice exams, including three take-home and two proctored tests. The instructors have a minimum of a master's degree and are experienced in teaching college-level courses.

PART V

beyond the mcat:

the medical school application process

Submit your application as early as possible.

A GREAT RELIEF comes from having completed the MCAT successfully. However, you should not celebrate too long and ignore other aspects of the application process. The American Medical College Application Service (AMCAS) begins to accept applications in mid-June. You would be well advised to submit your application as early as possible (e.g., by mid-July). Both the AMCAS and medical schools process applications on a rolling basis. Therefore, your file is evaluated in the order received. Medical schools do not wait to evaluate all the applicants before interviewing or even accepting students. This aspect is especially important for students who are borderline applicants; medical schools are more likely to grant interviews in the earlier months because of space availability. For example, a student with a 3.4 grade-point average (GPA) and a score of 10 on each section of the MCAT may be granted an interview at a school if 150 spaces are available but may not be when only 20 or fewer spaces are available later in the year. The same logic applies to competitive students who want to be accepted into competitive programs.

The Application

DO NOT BE INTIMIDATED. Just do it. Apply. For unknown reasons, some applicants cannot seem to get started with their applications. Remember: With the exception of the personal statement, this application is like most others. Writing your personal statement is, however, more complicated. Before you consult anyone, write out a few general topics that most admission committees want to know, for example, (1) why you want to become a doctor, (2) what your motivations are, (3) what significant events have occurred in your life, (4) your experience in a medical setting, (5) your research experience, and (6) your future goals. Initially, go for quantity, not quality. You may be surprised at how many pages you can fill. Next, hunt for personal statements from medical students, interns, residents, and others who may still have a copy of their application. Most people are happy to share them, and reading personal statements of successful applicants may be tremendously beneficial. Note, too, that not everything you wrote on your rough draft will fit on your final one-page application. But do not throw anything away; in a few weeks to months, you will be receiving secondary applications from medical schools requesting more information—in which case the additional thoughts on your rough drafts may be useful. Then, begin the most important task: edit, edit, and edit. Show the drafts to many people ahead of you in the game: advisors, medical students, residents, and a professional editor or English professor. Balance and integrate their feedback into something that reflects your personal strengths. Also remember that your personal statement reflects directly on you; therefore, it should be error-free. If you cannot make your page error-free get it professionally typed.

Choosing Where to Apply

CHOOSING THE SCHOOLS to which you will apply can be a difficult task. In general, applicants know their top few choices. However, you may not know how to choose the next group of schools (assuming you are applying to 30 schools). As mentioned earlier, this process is relatively expensive; therefore, you should take a few hours and go through the most recent *Medical School Admissions Requirements* book and *Curriculum Directory*, both published by AAMC. These two publications will give you a general idea about your chances for admission at specific schools (e.g., they will indicate that it is not wise to apply to a school in another state that accepts only its own students even if your GPA and MCAT score exceed their average). How many medical schools you should apply to depends on your goals and credentials, but applying to at least ten is reasonable.

Some candidates think that because they are strong applicants, they need apply only to the most competitive schools. This attitude is a mistake, because many "strong" applicants do not get into medical school for just this reason. Apply to some of the less competitive schools as "safe schools." Medical school admission committees are influenced by your acceptances to other schools. Besides, being accepted into even one medical school may give you a sense of relief, security, and self-confidence.

If you have been accepted by a medical school but you prefer another, let them know.

If you have been accepted to a medical school but you would prefer another, let that school know. Writing letters and making phone calls may be very useful. Remind the school of your existence and interest. If the school is nearby, it may be beneficial to visit. Remember: If you do not get accepted, you are no worse off than if you had not tried. If you are accepted, you may be in a better program or you may save thousands of dollars in the long run.

Letters of Recommendation

IN GENERAL, THE most important aspect of this part of the application process is to not let these letters delay the completion of your application. Letters of recommendation are usually similar. Some, however, make a student stand out for unique reasons (e.g., "This student is in the top 1% of all the students I have been associated with"); others are less than enthusiastic about a candidate (e.g., "He/she was a good student"). In such cases, the committee usually takes notice.

It may be difficult at the last moment to determine whom you want to write letters for you. You should plan ahead, even up to 1 to 3 years. It is important to get letters from people who know you well. Letters are usually obtained from research professors, hospital volunteer coordinators, instructors for classes in which you have done exceptionally well, leaders of other volunteer programs, and sometimes athletic directors.

Letters of recommendation should be requested several months in advance.

Requests for letters of recommendations should be made several months in advance of applying to medical schools. Generally, people writing these letters are even more busy than you are. Periodic reminders are helpful; however, there is a fine line between being persistent and being pushy. Do not rest until you know that your letters have been received either by the central processing agency at your university or by the programs that you have applied to. Applications have been known to be delayed several weeks to months because one or more letters had not been submitted (e.g., the professor went on vacation or letters were lost in mail or at the medical school admissions office). The bottom line is to plan ahead and keep on top of it.

The Interview

A few days before the interview, read about the school where you are interviewing.

MANY APPLICANTS FIND that interviews are the toughest part of the application process. However, this apprehension need not be a problem. Approximately 10% to 20% of medical school applicants are offered interviews. If you have been offered one, you have already crossed a major hurdle. Once again, preparation is the key. During the early part of the summer, even before you have been offered an interview, begin preparing. Videotape yourself during a mock interview with a counselor or a friend; you may be surprised by what you see, both good and bad. A few days before the interview, read about the school where you are interviewing, and learn its past, present, and future objectives. These objectives can be obtained from brochures or from students attending that school. Before the interview, review what is written on your personal statement. Many questions will come from that page.

keyword index